Intercollegiate MRCS:
Single Best Answer
Practice Papers

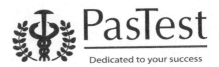

PasTest
Dedicated to your success

Intercollegiate MRCS: Single Best Answer Practice Papers

Irfan Halim
MBBS MRCS MSc
Specialist Registrar in General and
Laparoscopic Sugery
St George's Hospital Medical School
University of London

Kimberly Lammin
BSc MBChB MRCS
Specialist Registrar,
Trauma and Orthopaedics,
Royal Preston Hospital

Lorna Cook
BA MBBS MRCS
Clinical Fellow in General Surgery
Royal Sussex County Hospital, Brighton

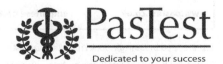

PasTest
Dedicated to your success

© 2006 PASTEST LTD

Egerton Court

Parkgate Estate

Knutsford

Cheshire

WA16 8DX

Telephone: 01565 752000

First Published 2006

ISBN: 1 904627 77 3

ISBN: 978 1 904627 77 7

A catalogue record for this book is available from the British Library.

The information contained within this book was obtained by the authors from reliable sources. However, while every effort has been made to ensure its accuracy, no responsibility for loss, damage or injury occasioned to any person acting or refraining from action as a result of information contained herein can be accepted by the publishers or authors.

PasTest Revision Books and Intensive Courses

PasTest has been established in the field of postgraduate medical education since 1972, providing revision books and intensive study courses for doctors preparing for their professional examinations.

Books and courses are available for the following specialties:

MRCGP, MRCP Parts 1 and 2, MRCPCH Parts 1 and 2, MRCPsych, MRCS, MRCOG Parts 1 and 2, DRCOG, DCH, FRCA, PLAB Parts 1 and 2, Dental Students, Dentists and Dental Nurses.

For further details contact:

PasTest, Freepost, Knutsford, Cheshire WA16 7BR

Tel: 01565 752000   **Fax: 01565 650264**

www.pastest.co.uk   **enquiries@pastest.co.uk**

Text prepared by Carnegie Book Production, Lancaster

Printed and bound in Great Britain by Antony Rowe Ltd, Chippenham, Wiltshire

Contents

Foreword

This book is intended primarily for candidates sitting the new MCQ section of MRCS Part 1 examination. The five practice papers included in this book each provide 90 questions in the new SBA or 'single best answer' format. Each of the papers has been specifically structured and the contents aim to reflect the syllabus as set by the Royal College of Surgeons.

The written component of the MRCS examination is set in Part 1 (MCQs), covering the applied basic sciences and Part 2 (EMQs), covering systematic clinical topics. This book aims to help you to pass the Part 1 MRCS examination: you will learn to assess your knowledge and also be alerted to those areas that may require further revision. This book alone is not a substitute for the necessary reading required before sitting the exam. It should be used in conjunction with a good background of reading materials that aim to cover the syllabus and other practice question books. The questions covered within these five practice papers represent a good range of 'hot-topics' that are found year to year within the MRCS examination. The questions are also set in levels of varying difficulty just as in the real exam. The answers include a paragraph justifying themselves as well as commenting on the relevant surgical topics.

I hope that you find this book helpful in guiding you in your future examinations. I hope also that this book will not be restricted to MRCS candidates, but be useful for Final Year medical students and other students of surgery.

Irfan Halim

Acknowledgements

I should like to make special mention of the following contributors who provided question material and expert advice for this book:

- Mr Scott Maskell (ENT)
- Mr Nirooshun Rajendran (GI Surgery)
- Mr Naveed Shaikh (Orthopaedics)
- Mr Ahmed Haq (Vascular)
- Mr Rene Chang (Transplant)
- Dr Kamal Halim (Pathology and Immunology)
- Mr Mumtazudeen Haider (GI Surgery)
- Miss Mehnaz Tawhid (Anatomy and Physiology)
- Mr Akash Sharma (Anatomy and Physiology)
- Mr Amir Halim (Paediatric Surgery)

Most importantly thanks are due to my wife Saila and my mum for helping me in just about every technical aspect of putting together a large part of this book. I would also to like thank my co-authors Kimberly Lammin and Lorna Cook in getting this book together to provide you with five complete MCQ practice papers for the new format SBA MRCS Part I examination.

Irfan Halim

Examination Technique

This is a brief guide which I hope you find helpful for the SBA paper of the MRCS.

Most of the points mentioned below are fairly obvious, but during the stress of the exam it is easy to forget some of them.

Revision
- Start revising early, you never have as much time as you thought you did
- Try and revise with someone else sitting the same exam
- Do plenty of practice questions so that you are familiar with the format

In The Exam Itself
- Read the instructions carefully
- Allow enough time to complete the paper
- If you are initially writing the answers on the question paper, make sure you allow time to transfer them to the answer sheet
- Always turn over the last page, you wouldn't be the first person to miss the last few questions
- Read the questions thoroughly paying particular attention to questions asking which of the following is correct/INcorrect
- If the question seems too simple, it probably is that straightforward, there should not be any trick questions in the exam

Good luck

Kim Lammin

Abbreviations

AAA	abdominal aortic aneurysm
ACE	angiotensin-converting enzyme
ACTH	adrenocorticotropic hormone
ADH	antidiuretic hormone
ALT	alanine aminotransferase
ANP	atrial natriuretic peptide
A–P	anteroposterior
APTT	activated partial thromboplastin time
ARDS	acute respiratory distress syndrome
ASA	American Society of Anaesthesiologists
ATLS	advanced trauma life support
BE	base excess
BMI	body mass index
BP	blood pressure
BPH	benign prostatic hypertrophy
BRCA1 and 2	familial breast cancer genes
C5a, C3a, C3b	complement functions
C1 to C7	cervical vertebrae
Ca	carcinoma
CABG	coronary artery bypass graft
cAMP	cyclic adenosine monophosphate
CEA	carcinoembryogenic antigen
CHARGE syndrome	coloboma and cranial nerve palsies; heart disease; atresia choana; retarded growth; genital abnormalities; ear abnormalities and deafness
CIN	cervical intraepithelial neoplasia
CMV	cytomegalovirus
COHb	carboxyhaemoglobin
COPD	chronic obstructive pulmonary disease
CRP	cAMP receptor protein

CSF	cerebrospinal fluid
CT	computed tomography
CVA	cerebrovascular accident
CVP	central venous pressure
CXR	chest X-ray
DCIS	ductal carcinoma in-situ
DIC	disseminated intravascular coagulation
2,3-DPG	2, 3-diphosphoglycerate
DPL	diagnostic peritoneal lavage
EBV	Epstein–Barr virus
ECF	extracellular fluid
ECG	electrocardiogram
Epo	erythropoietin
ERCP	endoscopic retrograde cholangiopancreatography
ESR	erythrocyte sedimentation rate
FAP	familial adenomatous polyposis
FFP	fresh frozen plasma
FiO_2	concentration of inspired oxygen
FNA	fine needle aspiration
FSH	follicle-stimulating hormone
5-FU	5-fluorouracil
G_0 to G_2 phase	phases in cell cycle
GCS	Glasgow Coma Scale
GFR	glomerular filtration rate
GGT	γ-glutamyltransferase
GH	growth hormone
GI	gastrointestinal
Hb	haemoglobin
HbF	fetal haemoglobin
HBV	hepatitis B virus
HCG	human chorionic gonadotropin
HER	Herceptin receptor
HIV	human immunodeficiency virus

HLA	human lymphocyte antigens
HNPCC	hereditary non-polyposis colon cancer
HR	heart rate
HTLV–1	human lymphocyte T-cell lymphotropic virus
Ig	immunoglobulin
ITU	intensive therapy unit
iu	international units
IV	intravenous
IVC	inferior vena cava
JVP	jugular venous pressure
KUB	kidney, ureter and bladder
L1 to L5	lumbar vertebrae
LDH	lactate dehydrogenase
LH	luteinising hormone
LH-RH	luteinising hormone-releasing hormone
LIMA	left internal mammary artery
LOAF	lumbricals, opponens pollicis, abductor pollicis brevis, flexor pollicis brevis muscles
M phase	phase in cell cycle
M0, M1	carcinoma stages (metastases)
MEN 1 & 2	multiple endocrine neoplasia syndromes
MI	myocardial infarction
MRI	magnetic resonance imaging
NADPH	[reduced form of] nicotinamide-adenine dinucleotide phosphate
N0, N1, N2, N3	carcinoma stages (nodes)
NEC	necrotising enterocolitis
NSGCT	non-seminomatous germ-cell tumour
NICE	National Institute for Health and Clinical Excellence
NK	natural killer
NSAID	non-steroidal anti-inflammatory drug
OGD	oesophago-gastro-duodenoscopy
PaO_2	partial pressure of oxygen
PAS	periodic acid–Schiff

PT	prothrombin time
pCO_2	partial pressure of carbon dioxide
PCWP	pulmonary capillary wedge pressure
PDS	polyglecapone polydioxanone sulphate
PPH	prolapse and haemorrhoidopexy
PPI	proton pump inhibitor
PR	per rectum
PSA	prostate-specific antigen
PTH	parathyroid hormone
PTFE	polytetrafluoroethylene (polytef)
PUJ	pelvi-ureteric junction
PUVA	psoralen plus ultraviolet A
Rb1	retinoblastoma
Rh	rhesus
RR	respiration rate
S phase	phase in cell cycle
S1 to S5	sacral vertebrae
SCC	squamous cell carcinoma
SFA	superficial femoral artery
SIRS	systemic inflammatory response syndrome
SLE	systemic lupus erytheromatosus
SVC	superior vena cava
T1, T2, T3, T4	carcinoma stages (tissues)
T1 to T12	thoracic vertebrae
T_3	tri–iodothyronine
T_4	thyroxine
TIA	transient ischaemic attack
Tis	in-situ carcinoma
TNM stages	tumour-node-metastases staging system
TPN	total parenteral nutrition
TSH	thyroid-stimulating hormone
TT	thrombin time
TUR	transurethral resection
TURP	transurethral resection of prostate

UC	ulcerative colitis
UTI	urinary tract infection
VHL	von Hippel–Lindau
VIN	vulvar intraepithelial neoplasia
VMA	vanillylmandelic acid
WCC	white cell count

PRACTICE PAPER 1: QUESTIONS

PRACTICE PAPER 1: QUESTIONS

1 **In the healthy full-term neonate, meconium should normally be passed**

○ A within 12 hours of birth

○ B within 24 hours of birth

○ C within 36 hours of birth

○ D within 48 hours of birth

○ E within the first 5 days

2 **Orchidopexy for undescended testes should be performed in children at which age?**

○ A immediately at diagnosis

○ B between 3 and 6 months of age

○ C between 6 and 12 months of age

○ D between 12 and 15 months of age

○ E any time before the onset of puberty

3   **The most common cause of childhood subglottic stenosis is**

- ○   A   congenital subglottic stenosis
- ○   B   gastro-oesophageal reflux
- ○   C   previous endotracheal tube intubation
- ○   D   previous tracheostomy
- ○   E   croup

4   **Which of the following are acceptable indications for performing an Emergency Room thoracotomy following chest trauma?**

- ○   A   haemothorax with an initial drainage of 1 L blood on chest tube drainage
- ○   B   continuing haemothorax of at least 100 mL/hour on chest tube drainage
- ○   C   presence of pulseless electrical activity following penetrating chest trauma
- ○   D   asystole following blunt chest trauma
- ○   E   worsening cardiac tamponade regardless of the nature of trauma

5   **All of the following are components of the Revised Trauma Scoring System with the exception of**

- ○   A   heart rate
- ○   B   respiratory rate
- ○   C   systolic BP
- ○   D   best verbal response to pain
- ○   E   best motor response to pain

6   An 18-year-old victim of a road traffic accident is brought into Casualty unconscious. She makes incomprehensible sounds and opens her eyes to pain. On further examination, her right arm extends when a painful stimulus is applied; however, her left arm localises to the area of discomfort. Her GCS score is

○   A   8

○   B   9

○   C   10

○   D   11

○   E   12

7   Absolute contraindications to DPL following major abdominal trauma include which one of the following

○   A   pregnancy

○   B   morbid obesity

○   C   evisceration of bowel

○   D   abdominal scarring from previous surgery

○   E   suspected internal bleeding

8   A 50 kg woman sustains full thickness burns to 40% of her body. Her fluid replacement for the next 8 hours will be

○   A   1600 mL

○   B   2800 mL

○   C   4000 mL

○   D   6600 mL

○   E   8000 mL

9   A 50-year-old woman complains of a cramping pain in her buttocks, which occurs after walking 50 yards and relieved by resting. You organise an angiogram to assess the pelvic and lower limb vasculature. Stenosis of which of the following vessels is suspected clinically?

- ⭘ A common iliac artery
- ⭘ B iliolumbar artery
- ⭘ C external iliac artery
- ⭘ D superficial femoral artery
- ⭘ E profunda femoris artery

10   A GP calls you for advice regarding a 80-year-old man who has a loud bruit in the right side of his neck. Outpatient Doppler investigations have revealed a 55% stenosis of the internal carotid artery. Appropriate advice on management of this man would include

- ⭘ A anti-platelet agents with lifestyle advice and treatment to control vascular risk factors
- ⭘ B urgent referral to a vascular surgeon
- ⭘ C elective endarterectomy
- ⭘ D elective bypass grafting
- ⭘ E observation alone as the patient is asymptomatic

11 **Thoracic outlet syndrome classically presents with all of the following EXCEPT**

○ A   neck and shoulder pain

○ B   digital gangrene owing to ischaemia

○ C   weakened radial pulse on arm elevation

○ D   wasting of the thenar eminence

○ E   paraesthesia along the ulnar border of the forearm

12 **A 33-year-old man presents with a month's history of foul-smelling creamy left ear discharge with some hearing loss and mild otalgia. On examination, there is a dark crusting mass overlying the pars flaccida. Rinne's test is negative on the left, and Weber's localises to the left. The diagnosis is**

○ A   otitis externa

○ B   cholesteatoma

○ C   canal exostoses

○ D   suppurative otitis media

○ E   glomus jugulare

13 **Which of the following statements is FALSE regarding laryngeal carcinoma?**

○ A   distant metastases are found in 20% of patients at presentation

○ B   squamous cell carcinoma of the larynx represents approximately 1% of malignancies in men

○ C   hoarseness is the commonest presenting symptom

○ D   verrucous carcinoma is a form of squamous cell carcinoma

○ E   the glottis has virtually no lymphatic drainage

14 **The initial drug of choice in the treatment of acute tonsillitis is**

○ A penicillin V

○ B ampicillin

○ C cefuroxime

○ D erythromycin

○ E metronidazole

15 **A 43-year-old man presents to the clinic with a slowly growing, painless firm mass antero-inferior to the left ear. He has no lymph nodes palpable. His facial movements are normal. The most likely diagnosis in this case is**

○ A Warthin's tumour

○ B salivary calculi

○ C mumps infection

○ D pleomorphic adenoma

○ E adenoid cystic carcinoma

16 **The following signs may be present in a tension pneumothorax EXCEPT with**

○ A hyper-resonance to percussion on the affected side

○ B increased elevated jugular venous pressure (JVP) on the opposite side

○ C tracheal shift to the affected side

○ D displaced apex beat

○ E absent breath sounds on the affected side

17   All of the following may be found in cardiac tamponade EXCEPT

○   A   widened pulse pressure

○   B   distended neck veins

○   C   hypotension

○   D   Kussmaul's sign

○   E   pulsus paradoxus

18   A 75-year-old man is brought into the Emergency Department with a 1-hour history of sudden onset severe chest pain radiating to the back, which occurred at rest. He has a history of rheumatoid arthritis, severe asthma, and hypertension. The heart rate is 105/min, BP is 170/95 mmHg and CXR shows a widened mediastinum. Appropriate management of this patient includes all of the following EXCEPT

○   A   insertion of large bore IV lines and fluid resuscitation

○   B   CT scan of the chest with contrast

○   C   initiation of intravenous beta blocker therapy

○   D   urgent referral to a cardiac surgeon

○   E   analgesia and medical management if a type B thoracic aortic dissection is found on investigation

19   Which of the following is not used in the management of an impacted food bolus in the oesophagus?

○   A   barium swallow

○   B   flexible nasendoscopy

○   C   buscopan

○   D   rigid oesophagoscopy

○   E   glucagon

20 A patient is referred to you in clinic with bilateral inguinal hernias. He is otherwise well. You advise him to have

- A bilateral open repair
- B unilateral open repair followed by the smaller hernia repaired at a later date
- C bilateral laparoscopic repair
- D a watch and wait for now
- E a truss

21 The following statements are true of gastric carcinoma in the UK EXCEPT

- A it is commoner in lower social classes
- B the site of cancer within the stomach moves more proximally with time
- C it is twice as common in men than women
- D it is rising in incidence
- E it is found most commonly in people with blood group A

22 The following are all components of the Glasgow prognostic criteria in assessing an attack of acute pancreatitis EXCEPT

- A white cell count
- B age
- C serum albumin levels
- D serum amylase levels
- E serum glucose levels

23   **A common complication following laparoscopic cholecystectomy is**

○   A   bowel perforation

○   B   capacitance coupling

○   C   common bile duct injury

○   D   shoulder tip pain

○   E   ileus

24   **A 31-year-old woman presents to you with recurrent abdominal pain and frequent bloody diarrhoea. You suspect inflammatory bowel disease and arrange for a colonoscopy with biopsy. Which one of the following features on biopsy would suggest ulcerative colitis (UC) over a diagnosis of Crohn's disease**

○   A   skip lesions

○   B   rosethorn ulceration

○   C   presence of granulomas

○   D   transmural (full thickness) involvement

○   E   presence of crypt abscesses

25   A 56-year-old man, who has recently had surgery for large bowel obstruction secondary to a pelvic mass, has had an erect CXR brought to your attention. His surgery was 3 days ago and he now appears to have an ileus but is comfortable. Free air is apparent under his diaphragm. His abdomen is distended and he is tender in the midline. The free air is likely to be due to

○   A   perforated bowel

○   B   a normal finding 3 days post laparotomy

○   C   an anastomotic breakdown

○   D   a diaphragmatic injury

○   E   perforated ulcer

26   A 68-year-old man presents with a rectal tumour palpable at approximately 10 cm from the anal verge. CT confirms this and the biopsy shows it to be a rectal adenocarcinoma. The best surgical option would be

○   A   a sigmoid colectomy

○   B   an A-P excision

○   C   an anterior resection

○   D   a left hemicolectomy

○   E   a subtotal colectomy

27   Right-sided tumours of the large bowel present more frequently with which of the following characteristics when compared to left-sided tumours?

○   A   large bowel obstruction

○   B   small bowel obstruction

○   C   blood mixed in with stools

○   D   change in bowel habit

○   E   iron-deficiency anaemia

28   Colonoscopy is indicated in all of the following people EXCEPT

○   A   a young brother of a patient with familial adenomatous polyposis (FAP)

○   B   a 52-year-old woman with unexplained iron deficiency anaemia

○   C   a 65-year-old patient with fresh PR bleeding from piles

○   D   a 45-year-old asymptomatic patient following removal of a hyperplastic polyp 1 year ago

○   E   a patient with curative resection of a caecal tumour by right hemicolectomy 2 years previously

29   A 62-year-old man presents to the hospital with large bowel obstruction. You decide to take this patient to the operating theatre after appropriate investigations and resuscitation. During laparotomy, a tumour is found in the transverse colon. Appropriate further management of this patient during surgery will include

○ A   transverse colectomy with defunctioning loop ileostomy

○ B   transverse loop colostomy

○ C   extended right hemicolectomy with defunctioning loop ileostomy

○ D   end ileostomy

○ E   left hemicolectomy with defunctioning loop ileostomy

30   All of the following statements regarding FAP are true EXCEPT

○ A   inheritance is autosomal dominant

○ B   the gene for FAP is carried on the short arm of chromosome 9

○ C   there is an association with congenital hypertrophy of the pigmented retina

○ D   all patients will eventually require a colectomy

○ E   OGD and sigmoidoscopy are always necessary in the postoperative surveillance period

31 **Advantages of the use of bipolar diathermy over monopolar include all of the following during surgery EXCEPT**

○ A   lack of pacemaker interference

○ B   not using the patient as part of an electrical circuit

○ C   avoidance of patient plate burns

○ D   avoidance of injuries from current channelling

○ E   ability to cut as well as coagulate

32 **All of the following are advantages of laparoscopic over open surgery EXCEPT**

○ A   reduced hospital stay

○ B   reduced operating time

○ C   earlier return to work

○ D   improved cosmesis

○ E   shorter recovery time

33 **Which one of the following is an absolute contraindication to performing laparoscopic surgery?**

○ A   pregnancy

○ B   BMI >40

○ C   previous abdominal surgery

○ D   having symptomatic chronic obstructive pulmonary disease (COPD)

○ E   presence of an uncorrected coagulopathy

34   All of the following are recognised clinical features of Horner's syndrome EXCEPT

○   A   ptosis

○   B   enophthalmos

○   C   meiosis

○   D   unilateral anhydrosis

○   E   Argyll Robertson pupil

35   A 27-year-old woman is undergoing a renal transplant from a cadaveric donor. Within minutes of the renal vessels being anastamosed, the kidney turns blue and becomes flaccid in nature. You diagnose hyperacute rejection on the basis that the histology shows deposition of immunoglobulins, complement, and neutrophils in the vessel walls. The immunological basis for this type of rejection is based on

○   A   preformed donor antibodies directed against the host antigens

○   B   preformed host antibodies directed against the donor antigens

○   C   donor cytotoxic T lymphocytes directed against host antigens

○   D   donor natural killer (NK) cells directed against host antigens

○   E   host NK cells directed against donor antigens

36   The following statements are true for squamous cell carcinoma (SCC) of the skin EXCEPT

○   A   xeroderma pigmentosum is a recognised risk factor

○   B   SCC occurs in sun exposed areas

○   C   SCC is called a Marjolin's ulcer when it occurs in chronic ulcers

○   D   metastases are more common in SCC than in basal cell carcinoma

○   E   psoralens appear to have a protective effect

37 Which of the following thyroid malignancies occurs most frequently?

○ A   papillary carcinoma (Ca)

○ B   follicular Ca

○ C   medullary Ca

○ D   anaplastic Ca

○ E   thyroid lymphoma

38 All of the following may found as part of the MEN 1 (multiple endocrine neoplasia) syndrome EXCEPT

○ A   gastrinoma

○ B   adrenal cortical adenoma

○ C   parathyroid hyperplasia

○ D   pituitary adenoma

○ E   phaeochromocytoma

39 A 20-year-old woman presents to the breast clinic with a firm painful 2 cm lump in the upper outer quadrant of the right breast. The lump is well-defined and extremely mobile. Your next step in managing this patient will be to

○ A   reassure and discharge if mammography is normal

○ B   observe in outpatient clinics and further investigate if there are any changes

○ C   perform an excision biopsy without the need for ultrasound

○ D   perform an ultrasound and excision biopsy without fine needle aspiration (FNA)

○ E   perform an ultrasound and FNA

40 **All of the following statements are true of solitary thyroid nodules EXCEPT**

○ A they are more prevalent in women

○ B in the adult population, more than 90% are benign

○ C they should be surgically removed in all patients

○ D less than 20% of cold nodules are malignant

○ E the risk of a hot nodule being malignant is very small

41 **The intercostal neurovascular bundle, which runs in the subcostal groove of the ribs, is located anatomically between which of the following layers?**

○ A between skin and subcutaneous tissues

○ B between subcutaneous tissues and the external intercostals

○ C between external intercostals and internal intercostals

○ D between internal intercostals and innermost intercostals

○ E between the innermost intercostals and the pleura

42 **Which of the following structures passing through the diaphragm are correctly associated with their corresponding vertebral levels?**

○ A T8 – oesophagus with vagus nerves

○ B T8 – aorta with the thoracic duct

○ C T10 – inferior vena cava (IVC) with the right phrenic nerve

○ D T10 – oesophagus with vagus nerves

○ E T10 – aorta with the thoracic duct

43   **The following arteries are all directly involved in the blood supply to the stomach EXCEPT**

○ A   right gastric artery

○ B   left gastric artery

○ C   gastroduodenal artery

○ D   short gastric arteries

○ E   left gastroepiploic artery

44   **The following layers are encountered when a standard muscle-splitting Lanz incision is made for appendicectomy EXCEPT**

○ A   Camper's fascia

○ B   external oblique aponeurosis

○ C   internal oblique muscle

○ D   rectus sheath

○ E   transversalis fascia

45   **Which of the following is true of the brachioradialis muscle?**

○ A   it originates from the lateral aspect of the supracondylar ridge of the radius

○ B   it is the main muscle involved in the supinator reflex

○ C   it attaches to the ulnar styloid process

○ D   it is supplied by the deep branch of the radial nerve

○ E   it may often contain a nerve supply from a branch of the musculocutaneous nerve

46 The lateral compartment of the leg is supplied by which of the following nerves?

○ A   tibial nerve

○ B   common peroneal nerve

○ C   lateral popliteal nerve

○ D   deep peroneal nerve

○ E   superficial peroneal nerve

47 A young boy has been stabbed in the right forearm. He now has difficulty in flexing his wrist and pronating the forearm along with loss of sensation over the lateral fingers on the palmar surface. Which of the following nerves has been injured?

○ A   deep branch of radial nerve

○ B   median nerve

○ C   ulnar nerve

○ D   superficial branch of radial nerve

○ E   median palmar nerve

48 Following pelvic surgery, a patient reports numbness along the medial thigh as well as weakness of hip adduction. Which nerve has most likely been injured during the operation?

○ A   obturator

○ B   femoral

○ C   inferior gluteal

○ D   superior gluteal

○ E   sciatic

49   The coronary sinus typically receives drainage from all of the
following cardiac veins EXCEPT the

- ○   A   great cardiac vein
- ○   B   anterior cardiac vein
- ○   C   middle cardiac vein
- ○   D   small cardiac vein
- ○   E   posterior cardiac vein

50   The afferent limb of the cremaster reflex is provided by which of
the following nerves?

- ○   A   genital branch of the genitofemoral nerve
- ○   B   femoral branch of the genitofemoral nerve
- ○   C   pudendal nerve
- ○   D   iliohypogastric nerve
- ○   E   ilio-inguinal nerve

51   All of the listed vessels contribute to Little's area in epistaxis
EXCEPT

- ○   A   sphenopalatine artery
- ○   B   superior labial artery
- ○   C   ascending pharyngeal artery
- ○   D   ophthalmic artery
- ○   E   anterior ethmoid artery

52   The diaphragm develops in utero with contributions from all of the following structures EXCEPT the

- ○   A   dorsal oesophageal mesentery
- ○   B   peripheral rim derived from the body wall
- ○   C   septum transversum
- ○   D   vertebromuscular ridges
- ○   E   pleuroperitoneal membranes

53   The manubriosternal angle (angle of Louis) is the anatomical landmark of all of the following EXCEPT

- ○   A   thoracic level T4
- ○   B   the level of the 2nd rib and costal cartilage
- ○   C   the level of the tracheal bifurcation (carina)
- ○   D   the level of the commencement of the arch of aorta
- ○   E   the level of T4 dermatome

54   In a study of heavy alcohol drinkers and chronic pancreatitis, the odds ratio is stated to be 0.2 (odds of having pancreatitis in those who drink heavily). This means that

- ○   A   for every five heavy drinkers, one will have chronic pancreatitis
- ○   B   for every five patients with pancreatitis, one will be a heavy alcohol drinker
- ○   C   for every six heavy drinkers, one will have chronic pancreatitis
- ○   D   for every six patients with pancreatitis, one will be a heavy alcohol drinker
- ○   E   it is difficult to make a conclusion and more data are needed

55 **Psammoma bodies are typically found in which of the following thyroid cancers?**

○ A papillary

○ B follicular

○ C medullary

○ D anaplastic

○ E lymphoma

56 **The following are all risk factors for vascular disease EXCEPT**

○ A homocystinaemia

○ B consumption of hard water

○ C familial dysbetalipoproteinaemia

○ D cigar smoking

○ E impaired glucose tolerance

57 **Flow within a vessel is directly affected by all of the following factors EXCEPT**

○ A radius of the vessel wall

○ B blood haematocrit

○ C length of the vessel

○ D vessel wall tension

○ E cardiac failure

58 Which of the following associations of hypersensitivity reactions with its corresponding disease is correct?

- A   type I – allergic contact dermatitis
- B   type II – pernicious anaemia
- C   type III – hyperacute renal graft rejection
- D   type IV – autoimmune haemolytic anaemia
- E   type V – Goodpasture's syndrome

59 Which one of the following disorders will cause hypercalcaemia?

- A   hypothyroidism
- B   hyperthyroidism
- C   myositis ossificans
- D   carcinoid syndrome
- E   acute pancreatitis

60 All of the following factors impair wound healing EXCEPT

- A   jaundice
- B   hypoglycaemia
- C   poor tissue oxygenation
- D   zinc deficiency
- E   presence of infection

61   Overwhelming post-splenectomy sepsis is most commonly due to which of the following organisms?

○   A   *Escherichia coli*

○   B   *Neisseria meningitidis*

○   C   *Streptococcus pneumoniae*

○   D   *Haemophilus influenzae*

○   E   *Staphylococcus aureus*

62   Donated blood is routinely screened for all of the following infections EXCEPT

○   A   hepatitis B

○   B   hepatitis C

○   C   HIV–2

○   D   syphilis

○   E   cytomegalovirus (CMV)

63   All of the following cause a shift of the oxygen dissociation curve to the right EXCEPT

○   A   increased temperature

○   B   increased pH

○   C   increased 2,3-DPG

○   D   increased pCO_2

○   E   lack of local tissue perfusion

64   A 25-year-old girl is diagnosed to have Cushing's disease secondary to an ACTH-secreting pituitary adenoma. Which of the following biochemical abnormalities would be expected on a blood test?

○   A   hyponatraemia

○   B   hypokalaemia

○   C   hypoglycaemia

○   D   hyperchloraemia

○   E   hypocalcaemia

65   The following are causes of metabolic acidosis with an increased anion gap EXCEPT

○   A   rhabdomyolysis

○   B   renal tubular acidosis

○   C   chronic diarrhoea

○   D   diabetic ketoacidosis

○   E   salicylate overdose

66   Which of the following electrolyte values are correctly associated with these IV fluid solutions?

○   A   0.9% normal saline – Na^+ 147 mmol/L

○   B   0.18% dextrose saline – Na^+ 25 mmol/L

○   C   Ringer's lactate – Na^+ 131 mmol/L

○   D   Hartman's solution – Na^+ 131 mmol/L

○   E   1.8% hypertonic saline – Na^+ 256 mmol/L

67   A 44-year-old woman undergoes resection of the terminal ileum for treatment of symptomatic Crohn's disease. She is at increased risk for which of the following diseases following surgery?

○   A   appendicitis

○   B   gastritis

○   C   cholecystitis

○   D   hepatitis

○   E   pancreatitis

68   The following physiological changes are seen in response to cardiogenic shock EXCEPT

○   A   ↑JVP

○   B   hypotension

○   C   cool peripheries

○   D   presence of a 3rd heart sound

○   E   decrease of the pulmonary capillary wedge pressure (PCWP)

69   Cerebral blood flow is increased in all of the following conditions EXCEPT during

○   A   systemic hypocarbia

○   B   seizures

○   C   systemic hypoxia

○   D   chronic anaemia

○   E   hypertension

70 **Raised serum amylase may be seen in all of the following conditions EXCEPT**

- ○ A   perforated duodenal ulcer
- ○ B   parotiditis
- ○ C   ruptured abdominal aortic aneurysm (AAA)
- ○ D   intestinal obstruction
- ○ E   hyperparathyroidism

71 **The characteristic features of a Colles' fracture include the following EXCEPT**

- ○ A   dinner fork deformity
- ○ B   radial displacement
- ○ C   occurring within 2.5 cm of wrist joint
- ○ D   subluxation of carpus
- ○ E   angulation in opposite direction to Smith's fracture

72   A 37-year-old man presents to the Casualty Department complaining of a painful, swollen and warm knee. There is no history of trauma. He feels unwell and his temperature is 38.5 degrees. He is unable to mobilise because of the pain. All of the following are correct steps in management of this patient in the emergency department EXCEPT

   A   an urgent full blood count with erythrocyte sedimentation rate (ESR) and cAMP receptor protein (CRP)

   B   high dose intravenous antibiotics

   C   knee X-ray

   D   analgesia

   E   blood cultures

73   Earliest pathological changes in bone during acute haematogenous osteomyelitis of childhood occur in the

   A   metaphyseal–physeal junction

   B   diaphysis

   C   metaphyseal–diaphyseal junction

   D   epiphysis

   E   subperiosteal portion of the metaphysis

74 **With regard to humeral supracondylar fractures**

○ A they most commonly occur in the elderly population

○ B the distal fragment is usually tilted forwards

○ C they should always be observed in theatre during daylight hours

○ D they require vigilant observation for signs of brachial artery damage

○ E reduction is helped by elbow extension with pressure applied behind the olecranon

75 **A 42-year-old man presents to A&E with a profusely bleeding scalp laceration acquired during a fall. You decide that he needs to have the laceration sutured under local anaesthetic. He has a past history of severe alcoholic cirrhosis and mild asthma. Which one of the following local anaesthetic agents is potentially toxic in this patient?**

○ A cocaine

○ B lignocaine (lidocaine)

○ C procaine

○ D benzocaine

○ E tetracaine

76   A 34-year-old woman is admitted to the neurosurgical unit with a large subarachnoid haemorrhage following rupture of a berry aneurysm. Appropriate management includes all of the following EXCEPT

○   A   early mobilisation

○   B   IV fluid rehydration

○   C   cerebral angiography within 24 hours of admission

○   D   initiation of nimodipine therapy

○   E   surgical clipping of the aneurysm following failed coiling

77   All of the following may be found in the transurethral resection (TUR) syndrome EXCEPT

○   A   hyponatraemia

○   B   tachycardia

○   C   confusion

○   D   nausea

○   E   hyperammoniaemia

78   Which one of the following types of renal stones is radiolucent on kidney, ureter and bladder (KUB) films?

○   A   calcium stones

○   B   struvite stones

○   C   urate stones

○   D   cystine stones

○   E   oxalate stones

79 Risk factors for bladder transitional cell carcinoma include all of the following EXCEPT

○ A smoking

○ B cyclophosphamide

○ C pelvic irradiation

○ D exposure to benzidine

○ E exposure to schistosomiasis

80 All of the following primary sites metastasise classically with osteolytic lesions EXCEPT

○ A kidney

○ B prostate

○ C breast

○ D lung

○ E thyroid

81 All of the following viruses have been directly linked to cancer pathogenesis EXCEPT

○ A herpes simplex virus

○ B hepatitis B virus

○ C human papilloma virus

○ D human lymphocyte T cell lymphotropic virus (HTLV-1)

○ E Epstein-Barr virus

82   **All of the following are prerequisites for screening tests to be valid EXCEPT**

○   A   natural history of the disease being screened for must be understood

○   B   results must always be audited

○   C   results of screening must always result in reduced morbidity and mortality

○   D   test must also be used to detect early recurrence as well as primary pathology

○   E   facilities for treatment MUST be made available

83   **Breast cancer is more commonly found in women who**

○   A   are multiparous

○   B   have an early menarche

○   C   live in a developing country

○   D   have an early menopause

○   E   have first pregnancy at an early age

84   **Which one the following is correctly a component of the definition of SIRS (systemic inflammatory response syndrome)?**

○   A   heart rate >100/min

○   B   temperature <35°C or >38°C

○   C   respiratory rate >25/min

○   D   partial pressure of carbon dioxide (pCO_2) <32 mmHg

○   E   white cell count (WCC) >4000 or <11,000, or >10% immature forms

85 **Which of the following features of bowel ischaemia suggest a high mortality?**

○ A   haemorrhagic free fluid at laparoscopy

○ B   low oxygen saturation on blood gas

○ C   presence of atrial fibrillation

○ D   serum lactate >4 mmol/L

○ E   white cell count (WCC) $>20 \times 10^9$

86 **Evidence-based treatments proven in managing ARDS (acute respiratory distress syndrome) include all of the following EXCEPT**

○ A   early steroid administration

○ B   prone position ventilation

○ C   activated protein C

○ D   inverse ratio ventilation

○ E   inhaled nitric oxide

87 **You wish to proceed with organ donation from a patient with a severe spinal cord and head injury and suspected brainstem death. All of the following criteria may be used in the diagnosis of brainstem death following injury EXCEPT**

○ A   absence of the pupillary light reflex

○ B   absence of the corneal reflex

○ C   absence of the gag and cough reflex

○ D   absence of limb spinal reflexes

○ E   absence of motor cranial nerve function

88   Complications of massive blood transfusion include all of the
following EXCEPT

○   A   hypothermia

○   B   hyperthermia

○   C   hyperkalaemia

○   D   hypercalcaemia

○   E   metabolic acidosis

89   A 50-year-old man is admitted to the hospital to undergo an
anterior resection for carcinoma of the rectum. He has a long
history of asthma and has been taking 5 mg prednisolone for the
previous 3 months since his last discharge from hospital following
an acute attack. Which of the following steroid replacement
regimens is ideal in this patient?

○   A   50 mg hydrocortisone IV preoperatively only

○   B   50 mg hydrocortisone IV preoperatively and 6 hourly for the first
24 hours

○   C   100 mg hydrocortisone IV preoperatively and then 50 mg
6 hourly for at least the first 48 hours

○   D   100 mg hydrocortisone IV preoperatively and then 100 mg
6 hourly for at least the first 48 hours

○   E   100 mg hydrocortisone IV preoperatively and then 100 mg
6 hourly for at least the first 72 hours

90   A 67-year-old woman is admitted to the hospital for a total hip
replacement. Her past medical history includes a single
myocardial infarction (MI) which occurred 2 years ago, stable
angina controlled with tablets, hypertension, insulin dependent
diabetes and a previous renal transplant. Her ASA class is

○   A   ASA 1

○   B   ASA 2

○   C   ASA 3

○   D   ASA 4

○   E   ASA 5

PRACTICE PAPER 1: ANSWERS AND TEACHING NOTES

PRACTICE PAPER 1: ANSWERS AND TEACHING NOTES

1   B

The first stool is passed within 24 hours of birth in 99% of healthy full-term infants and within 48 hours in all healthy full-term infants. Failure of a full-term newborn to pass meconium within the first 24 hours should raise a suspicion of intestinal obstruction. Lower intestinal obstruction may be associated with disorders such as Hirschsprung's disease, anorectal malformations, meconium plug syndrome, small left colon syndrome, hypoganglionosis, and neuronal intestinal dysplasia.

2   D

Undescended testes should undergo further examination and orchidoplexy between 12 and 15 months of age. There is evidence of early damage to sperm-producing germ cells as well as an increased risk of carcinoma in later life for undescended testes.

3   C

Subglottic stenosis is acquired in 95% of cases, and 90% of these are due to previous intubation. Only 5% of stenoses are due to congenital causes. The most important risk factor is duration of intubation. Other causes include trauma, post-surgical trauma, such as previous cricothyroidotomy or high tracheostomy. Gastro-oesophageal reflux may worsen pre-existent subglottic stenosis, or be a factor in its own right in patients with no previous history of endotracheal intubation or laryngotracheal trauma. Croup causes subglottic swelling and will be worse in patients with pre-existent subglottic stenosis.

4   C

Emergency room thoracotomy should be performed only by a qualified surgeon. The indications are for penetrating trauma only where the patient undergoes a witnessed arrest that is not asystole. Initial drainage of >1.5 L of blood or continued drainage of >200 mL/hour are also indications for thoracotomy; however, it usually can be done in theatres while the patient is resuscitated en-route.

Pericardiocentesis can be performed for pericardial tamponade in the initial setting.

5   A

Components of the Revised Trauma Scoring System include respiratory rate, systolic BP, and Glasgow Coma Scale score, but not heart rate.

6   B

Eyes open to pain = 2

Localises pain = 5

Makes incomprehensible sounds = 2

Therefore GCS = 9

7   C

The only absolute contraindication to DPL is the need for laparotomy. Of the listed conditions, only evisceration of bowel necessitates laparotomy. The other conditions listed are relative contraindications.

8   C

The ATLS guideline for fluid resuscitation in burns states that ideally 2–4 mL/kg/% burns should be given in the first 24 hours. Half of this should be given in the first 8 hours. The higher fluid volume of 4 mL/kg/% burns should be used for full thickness burns as there is less of a skin barrier. Also the aim is to minimise renal failure from myoglobinuria and keep the kidney well flushed.

9   A

Buttock claudication should alert the clinician to suspect a stenosis of either the internal iliac artery or common iliac artery. External iliac artery or profunda femoris stenosis would cause thigh claudication. Superficial femoral artery (SFA) stenosis classically causes calf claudication.

Buttock claudication and impotence in males should raise suspicion of Leriche's syndrome, which is due to internal iliac stenosis.

10   A

Asymptomatic carotid artery stenosis which is <70% stenosed should be managed conservatively with antiplatelet agents such as aspirin and changes in lifestyle measures along with risk reduction strategies.

11   D

The commonly affected roots in thoracic outlet syndrome include the C8 and T1 roots resulting in wasting of hypothenar muscles as well as medial forearm. Although there are reported cases of median nerve involvement in severe cases, this is not classical of the syndrome generally.

12   B

A cholesteatoma is a three-dimensional epidermal structure made of keratinising squamous cells, exhibiting independent growth replacing middle ear mucosa and resorbing underlying bone. It is due to implanted epithelium. It produces a discharge, often foul and creamy. Deafness can be conductive from ossicular erosion, or sensory via toxin production. Attic crusting, marginal perforations, or debris containing retraction pockets are the principal signs. A rounded pearly white mass is diagnostic. Otitis externa affects just the external canal. Canal exostoses are external canal hyperostoses. Suppurative otitis media presents with an erythematous bulging tympanic membrane. Glomus jugulare is a rare hypervascular tumour that arises within the jugular foramen of the temporal bone.

13   A

Squamous cell carcinoma of the larynx represents approximately 1% of malignancies in men. It is five times commoner in men than women. Smoking tobacco and drinking alcohol predisposes towards carcinoma. Hoarseness is the commonest and maybe the only presenting symptom. Stridor and dyspnoea are late symptoms. Verrucous carcinoma is a variant of well-differentiated squamous cell carcinoma. Tumours affecting just the glottis have minimal risk of metastases as there is virtually no glottic lymphatic drainage. Metastases normally imply spread into adjacent sites such as the subglottis or supraglottis.

14   A

Most acute tonsillitis is caused by viral infections in up to 50% of occasions. Penicillin V is the drug of choice as most bacterial tonsillitis is caused by penicillin-sensitive Group A beta haemolytic streptococci. Ampicillin should never be used in acute tonsillitis as this causes generalised maculopapular rash in patients with wrongly diagnosed infectious mononucleosis. Erythromycin is given to patients allergic to penicillin.

15   D

The parotid is affected by 80% of all salivary tumours: 80% of parotid tumours are benign and 80% of benign tumours in the parotid gland are pleomorphic adenomas. Gender incidence is equal and occurs most commonly in the fifth decade. Management involves superficial parotidectomy; recurrence is possible. Warthin's tumour (papillary cystadenoma) is a benign tumour seen in elderly men in their seventh decade. Adenoid cystic carcinoma is the commonest malignant tumour, commonly in minor glands. Patients often complain of facial pain and may present with facial paresis. Mumps infection often causes bilateral parotitis in young patients. Salivary calculi are commonest in submandibular glands, owing to higher concentrations of mucus. Swelling and pain occurs on eating.

16   C

A tension pneumothorax presents with acute dyspnoea and occasionally chest pain. This may lead to sudden collapse, and an urgent pleural decompression is required to prevent cardiorespiratory compromise. The signs include decreased breath sounds and hyper-resonance to percussion on the affected side along with a tracheal shift to the opposite side. Displacement of the apex beat may occur with mediastinal shift, and the JVP would be raised bilaterally as the thoracic pressure is increased.

17   A

Cardiac tamponade is a medical emergency where fluid or blood may accumulate within the pericardial space and compress the heart resulting in failure of the cardiac pump. This is similar to a tension pneumothorax and can present with sudden collapse or deterioration in cardiac function. Signs include muffled heart sounds on auscultation, hypotension, narrowed pulse pressure, low voltage ECG complexes, raised JVP, Kussmaul's sign, and pulsus paradoxus. An urgent pericardiocentesis should relieve the pressure from within the enclosed pericardial space.

18   C

Ideally, the management of a thoracic dissection should be to resuscitate the patient as soon as possible and to decide on a management plan. Investigations are ideal when the patient is stable. Most type B dissections are medically manage with control of hypertension; however, in this case, the patient suffers from severe asthma, so IV β-blocker therapy is contraindicated. Other antihypertensive measures should be used in the meanwhile and a cardiac surgeon should be involved in the decision making as soon as possible.

19   A

Impaction of foreign bodies depends on their size and shape. Aerodigestive tract abnormalities make impaction more likely. Assessment is initially via plain lateral and anteroposterior neck and chest radiographs. Flexible nasendoscopy may demonstrate impaction at the cricopharyngeus. Barium swallow is not used as it coats the mucosa making oesophagoscopy and identification of a foreign body difficult. IV buscopan and diazepam is often used as first line. Studies have shown glucagon to aid in oesophageal sphincter relaxation. Failure to pass conservatively will require removal via rigid oesophagoscopy under general anaesthesia.

20   C

NICE guidelines suggest the use of laparoscopic surgery for the treatment of bilateral inguinal hernias. In centres where this is not performed, the open approach must be employed however, given the choice, the laparoscopic surgeon should be advised.

21   D

Gastric cancer has declined in incidence over the last century. It is twice as common in men and commoner in lower social classes, Japanese people, and persons with blood group A. Other risk factors include dietary nitrosamines, pernicious anaemia, post-gastrectomy, atrophic gastritis, hypogamma-globulinaemia, and presence of *Helicobacter pylori*. Interestingly, over the last half century, the site of gastric cancer has moved more proximally.

22   D

Glasgow (Imrie) scoring system for acute pancreatitis includes:
One point for each of the following: age >55; WBC >15 × 10^9; glucose >10 mmol/L; urea >16 mmol/L; PaO$_2$ <8 kPa; calcium <2 mmol/L; albumin <32 g/L; LDH >600 iu/L, ALT >100 iu/L. Any score >3 constitutes a severe attack of acute pancreatitis.

23   D

Shoulder tip pain is a common sequelae to laparoscopic surgery. This occurs as the diaphragm undergoes irritation from the excess gas in the peritoneal cavity. The referred pain travels along the phrenic nerve route and is referred to the shoulder tip quite commonly. The other listed complications are recognised but uncommon.

24   E

The presence of crypt abscess on biopsy is suggestive of ulcerative colitis (UC). Crohn's disease shows the presence of skip lesions with thickening of the bowel wall including encroachment onto mesenteric fat. A linear mucosal ulceration is also seen on macroscopic appearance leading to a 'cobblestone' pattern of islands of surviving mucosa. UC reveals an inflamed and ulcerated mucosal pattern that exhibits contact bleeding and is continuous from the rectum proximally. Fistulae may occur in Crohn's but not UC.

25   B

The presence of free intraperitoneal air is common following any intra-abdominal surgery, whether open or laparoscopic. Other causes include perforation of a viscus, the presence of gas-forming organisms, or even following waterskiing in women where air enters via the genital tracts. Free air takes a few days to resolve provided the original pathology or procedure has been dealt with, and absorption is usually complete within 5 days.

26   C

Anterior resections are performed for rectal cancers, which can be excised adequately with a sufficient anorectal margin distally. For the very distal rectal tumours or anal tumours, an abdominoperineal resection must be undertaken with an end stoma.

Sigmoid colectomies can be used for treatment of sigmoid tumours or excision of an area of diverticular disease, and left hemicolectomies for left colonic tumours.

27   E

Right-sided tumours more frequently present with iron deficiency, as their symptoms may be masked simply by their location within the GI tract. An obstructive presentation is less likely than left-sided tumours because the colonic contents are virtually liquid as they enter the ileocaecal junction and hence pass through even tight malignant strictures on the right side. For a similar stenosis on the left side, a faecal bolus may impact and present with obstruction. Also, blood is more noticeable on the stools for left-sided tumours as is a change in bowel habit.

28   D

Hyperplastic polyps generally do not require any colonoscopic follow-up as they are benign lesions. Certainly in an asymptomatic 45-year-old, a repeat colonoscopy is not warranted 1 year later. Other indications for colonoscopy include the investigation of PR bleeding, change in bowel habit, unexplained iron deficiency anaemia, follow-up post-cancer surgery, and for a strong family history as a risk factor.

29   C

Transverse colon tumours are best treated with an extended right hemicolectomy and a defunctioning loop ileostomy to protect the anastomosis, as oedamatous bowel from the obstruction may weaken the join. Transverse colectomies are inferior to extended right hemicolectomies: studies have revealed that a more complete lymph node dissection can occur with taking the right colic nodes as part of the right hemicolectomy as well as making a superior anastomosis from the ileocolic join as opposed to the colo-colic join.

30   B

FAP is an autosomal dominant condition leading to adenomatous polyps in the large bowel from the second decade onwards. The gene for FAP is carried on the long arm of chromosome 5. FAP is associated with congenital hypertrophy of the retinal pigment epithelium and gastroduodenal polyps, hence the need for lifelong OGD [AQ] even after a mandatory prophylactic colectomy has been performed.

31   E

Bipolar diathermy uses the principle of high current channelling, which occurs between the two tips of the diathermy forceps to coagulate tissue only. Cutting is accomplished by the use of monopolar diathermy in which the patient is used as part of a circuit, and can be complicated by diathermy plate burns, pacemaker interference, and current channelling in the digits or peripheries.

32   B

Laparoscopic surgery has its advantages over open surgery with improved cosmesis leading to an earlier recovery and shorter postoperative hospital stay, reduced pain, and an earlier return to work after surgery. The operating time is variable, but in most procedures it is longer than the open time.

33   E

The presence of an uncorrected coagulopathy is a contraindication to any surgical procedure. A BMI >40, pregnancy, previous abdominal surgery, and other systemic disorders are relative contraindications; however, recently surgeons have taken on board such cases without problem. A BMI >40 is the norm for most laparoscopic bariatric surgeons.

34   E

An Argyll–Robertson pupil is a small, irregular pupil that does not react to light but does react to accommodation. It is seen in cases of tertiary syphilis. Horner's syndrome is characterised by the presence of ptosis, miosis, enophthalmos, and anhidrosis.

35   B

The clinical scenario presented here is that of a hyperacute rejection. This type of rejection occurs on table immediately during the transplant itself after vascularisation of the kidney has been achieved, and is immunologically due to preformed host antibodies directed against the donor antigens.

36   E

Psoralens and psaloren plus ultraviolet A (PUVA) treatment increase the risk of developing squamous cell carcinoma (SCC) of the skin. Other risk factors include frequent exposure to sunlight over many years, fair skin, blond hair, blue eyes, family history, sensitive skin, chronic ulcers, actinic keratoses, radiation, arsenic/coal/tar exposure, immunosuppression, tobacco use, xeroderma pigmentosum, and previous SCC of the skin.

37   A

Papillary carcinomas are the most frequent of all the thyroid malignancies comprising 60–80% of all thyroid malignancies. Follicular carcinomas (10–18%), medullary carcinomas (5–10%), thyroid lymphomas (<2%), and anaplastic carcinomas (5–15%) occur less commonly.

38   E

Phaeochromocytomas are found as part of the MEN 2 syndrome. MEN 1 comprises parathyroid, pituitary, and pancreatic neoplasms. Occasionally, adrenal cortical adenomas may also occur as part of the MEN 1 syndrome.

39 D

A young woman presenting with a well-defined mobile breast lump is clinically presenting with a fibroadenoma. Although this may be left alone as it is a benign condition, ideally a histological diagnosis should be obtained for completeness. This is best done by excising the lump and will also provide reassurance and peace of mind to the patient that the lump has been removed. An FNA may be inconclusive and a histological diagnosis is better than a cytological one. An ultrasound is done at the same time to further assess the lump architecture and look for other co-existing lumps that may be removed at the same time.

40 C

Nodules detected by thyroid scans are classified as cold, hot or warm: 85% of thyroid nodules are cold, 10% are warm, and 5% are hot. Also remember that 85% of cold nodules are benign, 90% of warm nodules are benign, and 95% of hot nodules are benign. They are about four more times commoner in women. Not all thyroid nodules require excision, especially if they are asymptomatic and may be treated conservatively.

41 D

The intercostals neurovascular bundle runs in the subcostal groove under each rib and consists of a vein, artery, and nerve running superiorly to inferiorly. This bundle is located between the internal and innermost intercostals muscular layers.

42   D

The following structures pass through the main openings in the diaphragm:

T8 – IVC and right phrenic nerve

T10 – oesophagus with right and left vagus nerve, left gastric artery and vein, and lymphatics

T12 – Aorta, thoracic duct, and azygos vein.

43   C

The blood supply to the stomach is entirely derived from the coeliac axis. The following arteries directly supply the stomach:

- short gastric arteries – fundus
- right and left gastric arteries – lesser curvature
- right and left gastroepiploic arteries – greater curvature

The gastroduodenal artery runs behind the first part of the oesophagus and divides into the right gastroepiploic and superior pancreaticoduodenal arteries.

44   D

The Lanz incision incises through the skin, subcutaneous tissue, external oblique aponeurosis, internal oblique muscle (split), transversus abdominis, extraperitoneal fat, and peritoneum. The rectus muscle and sheath are encountered if the incision is too medially placed, but should not be encountered in a standard Lanz incision.

45   B

The brachioradialis muscle is the main muscle involved in the so-called 'supinator' reflex. It arises from the upper two-thirds of the lateral supracondylar ridge of the humerus and inserts into the radial styloid process. It is supplied by the main radial nerve and is involved in flexion of the elbow in a semi-prone position.

46   E

The lateral compartment of the leg comprises the peroneus longus and brevis muscles, both of which evert the ankle at the sub-talar joint. They are both supplied by the superficial peroneal nerve.

47   B

The median nerve can be injured in stab wounds to the anterior cubital fossa along with the brachial artery. Damage to this nerve at the elbow results in loss of pronation, weakness of wrist flexion with deviation, and loss of sensation on the lateral palm and radial three and a half digits.

48   A

The adductors of the hip are supplied by the obturator nerve, which arises from the anterior primary rami of L2, L3 and L4. The skin overlying the medial compartment of the thigh is also supplied by this nerve. Damage is not a common occurrence, but can occur with deep pelvic dissection, especially deep and medial to the inferior aspect of the psoas muscle.

49   B

The anterior cardiac veins drain directly into the anterior aspect of the right atrium. The other listed veins drain directly into the coronary sinus. The posterior cardiac vein may occasionally join the great cardiac vein instead of direct drainage into the sinus.

50   B

The cremasteric reflex is mediated by the two branches of the genitofemoral nerve. The afferent limb of this reflex is mediated by the femoral branch of the genitofemoral nerve and the efferent limb by the genital branch.

51   C

Little's area (also known as Kiesselbach's plexus) is implicated in anterior epistaxis. It is located over the anterior nasal septum and is formed by anastamoses between the sphenopalatine, greater palatine, superior labial, and anterior ethmoid arteries (which is a branch of the ophthalmic artery). These are branches of both the external and internal carotids. The ascending pharyngeal artery anastomoses with the posterior nasal and sphenopalatine vessels over the posterior middle turbinate in an area known as Woodruff's plexus. This area is implicated in posterior epistaxis.

52   D

The diaphragm develops in utero receiving contributions from the four following structures:

- dorsal oesophageal mesentery
- peripheral rim derived from the body wall
- septum transversum
- pleuroperitoneal membranes.

It develops cranially and acquire its cervical nerve supply from the phrenic nerve (C3, 4, 5), and migrates caudally to lie between the thorax and abdomen.

53   E

The manubriosternal angle of Louis marks the level of the second costal cartilage and rib. It is situated about the level of T4/T5 and is anatomically related to the level of the tracheal bifurcation and commencement of the aortic arch. The T4 dermatome is classically marked by the internipple line.

54   C

The odds in heavy drinkers of having chronic pancreatitis is quoted as 0.2 or 1/5. This means that for every one heavy drinker with the disease, five heavy drinkers will not (ie 1 out of every 6 heavy drinkers will be affected).

55   A

Pathologically, a psammoma body is a round, collection of calcium, seen on microscopy. The term is derived from the Greek word *psammos* meaning 'sand'. They are theoretically supposed to originate from a single necrotic cell in which layers of calcium salts are deposited. Psammoma bodies may be found in papillary thyroid, endometrial ovarian adenocarcinomas, meningiomas and mesotheliomas.

56   B

Drinking hard water has shown to have a protective effect in preventing vascular disease and the converse is true for soft water, which is a risk factor. High levels of blood homocysteine and hyperlipidaemia are other risk factors for vascular disease.

57   D

Poiseuille's law states that the flow within a vessel is directly proportional to the radius to the power of 4 and inversely proportional to the viscosity of the blood (including haematocrit) and length of the vessel. Flow will also be affected in cardiac pump failure, but not directly by vessel wall tension.

58   B

Hypersensitivity type I – immediate hypersensitivity or allergy

Hypersensitivity type II – antibody to cell bound antigen (cytotoxic)

Hypersensitivity type III – immune complex reaction

Hypersensitivity type IV – delayed hypersensitivity

Hypersensitivity type V – IgG Ab stimulatory effect.

59   B

Hyperthyroidism is a recognised cause of hypercalcaemia. This is thought to be due to a direct effect of the thyroid hormone primarily on bone metabolism; however, the exact mechanism is still unclear.

60   B

Local factors that impair wound healing include poor blood supply, haematoma, infection, early movement, foreign bodies, radiation, and denervation. Systemic factors include malnutrition and zinc/vitamin C deficiency, drugs, neoplasia, diabetes, older age, jaundice, and uraemia. Hyperglycaemia from diabetes as opposed to hypoglycaemia would impair wound healing.

61   C

Overwhelming post-splenectomy sepsis is due to infection with encapsulated organisms, the most common being *Streptococcus pneumoniae*. Patients are also at risk from *Haemophilus influenzae* and *Neisseria meningitidis* infections but to a lesser extent than from streptococcal infections.

62   E

Blood from donors in the UK is not routinely screened for CMV unless it is used for donation in special groups such as neonates and immunosuppressed patients. Screening does occur for syphilis (treponema), HIV, hepatitis B and hepatitis C.

63   B

A right shift in the oxygen dissociation curve decreases oxygen affinity allowing oxygen to be released only at higher partial pressures. This is known as the Bohr effect and the mechanism serves to increase oxygen extraction. Causes of right shift include acidosis, increased temperature, and increased levels of 2,3-DPG in the blood.

64   B

Cushing's disease will cause a hypokalaemia, along with hypernatraemia and hyperglycaemia owing to the excess cortisol secreted from the adrenal cortex or endogenous sources.

65   C

The normal anion gap is 10–16 mmol/L. It is calculated by subtracting the difference between the cations (Na and K) and anions (HCO_3 and Cl). It reflects the presence on unmeasured anions in the serum and will be raised in the presence of lactate, ketones, or other ingested agents such as aspirin in overdose. Chronic diarrhoea results in a loss of bicarbonate; however, this is matched by a compensatory increase in serum Cl so that the anion gap remains normal.

66   D

Hartman's solution contains 131 mmol/L of Na^+

0.9% normal saline contains 154 mmol/L of Na^+

0.18% saline contains 30 mmol/L

Ringer's lactate contains 147 mmol/L Na^+.

67   C

Terminal ileal resection due to Crohn's disease leads to loss of bile salt reabsorption. Hence, these patients have an increased cholesterol secretion and a lowered bile acid secretion, which leads to cholesterol supersaturation and the formation of gallstones.

68   E

Cardiogenic shock is a major complication of a variety of acute and chronic disorders that impair the ability of the heart to maintain adequate tissue perfusion. This most commonly follows acute myocardial infarctions. Haemodynamic criteria include sustained hypotension, reduced cardiac index, and an elevated pulmonary capillary wedge pressure (PCWP). Bedside signs may include cool peripheries, gallop rhythm, elevated JVP, low pulse pressure, and distant heart sounds.

69   A

Cerebral blood flow is increased in seizures, systemic hypoxia and hypercarbia, chronic anaemia, and hypertension. Hypocarbia causes cerebral vasoconstriction and reduced blood flow.

70   E

Raised serum amylase is classically seen in acute pancreatitis.
Other causes include:

- **congenital** – congenital hyperamylasaemia
- **acquired** – infection, eg mumps
  - neoplasm, eg pancreatic carcinoma
  - vascular, eg mesenteric ischaemia
  - inflammatory, eg hepatitis, post-ERCP (endoscopic retrograde cholangiopancreatography), peritonitis
  - trauma, eg burns, perforated duodenal ulcer, intestinal obstruction or perforation
  - drugs, eg opiates
  - metabolic, eg renal failure, renal transplant, diabetic ketoacidosis, macroamylasaemia.

71   D

Dinner fork deformity, radial displacement, and a fracture within 2.5 cm of the wrist joint are characteristic of a Colles' fracture, as well as radial shortening. There is commonly an associated ulnar styloid fracture. Carpal subluxation usually occurs when there is a Barton's fracture (intra-articular fracture through the dorsal or volar lip of the distal radius). Smith's fracture is an extra-articular fracture with volar displacement.

72   B

The clinical picture is of septic arthritis. The correct management of this presentation should be a thorough history and examination. A full blood count and inflammatory markers should be obtained to ascertain the extent of sepsis and because they are helpful for suture monitoring. Blood cultures can be positive, especially when taken during a period of pyrexia. The knee should be aspirated with an aseptic technique in clean surroundings, ie in theatre and NOT the casualty department. Only after the samples for microbiology have been obtained can the patient be given antibiotics. Knee X-rays will rule out bony pathology and can act as a baseline if there is joint destruction in the future.

73   A

The vascularity in the region of the metaphyseal–physeal junction is the greatest and therefore this area is affected first in osteomyelitis. Infection spreads to the subperiosteal and diaphyseal areas afterwards. The epiphysis is affected early in the presence of septic arthritis.

74   D

Supracondylar fractures are commoner in children. Falling onto an outstretched hand hyperextends the child's elbow leading the distal fragment to tilt posteriorly. The anteriorly tilted proximal fragment can damage the brachial artery. Such cases of supracondylar fractures should be taken to theatre as soon as possible as delay leads to excessive swelling and difficulty in reduction. Reduction is performed by flexing the elbow and applying pressure behind the olecranon.

75   B

Amide-type local anaesthetics such as lignocaine undergo hydrolysis by microsomal enzymes in the liver. The metabolism of such types of anaesthetics can be affected by severe liver dysfunction and are best avoided in such cases. Ester-type local anaesthetics are mainly hydrolysed by pseudocholinesterases.

76   A

Subarachnoid haemorrhage represents a neurosurgical emergency. It may be caused by trauma or spontaneously occur when a berry aneurysm ruptures leading to haemorrhage. Management includes early referral to a neurosurgical unit for bed rest, IV fluids, nimodipine therapy, cerebral angiography and coiling of the aneurysm. Other alternatives include clipping of the aneurysm base through open surgery and insertion of a ventricular drain to allow any blood to drain out and prevent a hydrocephalus from forming.

77   B

TUR syndrome results from hypervolaemia owing to excessive absorption of irrigation fluid during transurethral resections. A dilutional hyponatraemia results, with bradycardia and hypotension. Confusion and hyperammonaemia may be seen if metabolism of absorbed glycine from the irrigation fluid occurs. Management of this condition includes stopping the irrigation fluid, administering diuretics, and possibly twice normal saline as well. It is advisable to seek senior advice early on in this situation.

78   C

Over 90% of renal calculi are radio-opaque. Urate or uric acid stones arise in acidic urine and are generally hard light-brown stones which are smooth on the surface with facets.

79   E

Schistosomiasis is a risk factor for squamous and not transitional cell carcinoma of the bladder, which occurs more commonly in clinical practice. Other risk factors for transitional cell carcinoma include smoking, irradiation, drugs such as cyclophosphamide, exposure to chemical substances such as benzidine and β-naphthylamine; dyes used in textile, printing, and rubber industries.

80   B

The commonest of tumours to metastasise to bone include kidney, prostate, breast, lung, and thyroid tumours. Most of these form osteolytic bony metastases with the exception of prostate cancers which cause a sclerotic lesion most commonly in the lumbar spine, as the venous drainage via Batson's plexus is connected.

81   A

Herpes simplex virus has not yet been identified as a cancer-causing virus. It is associated with high-risk infectious groups who may also carry the hepatitis, HIV, and human papilloma viruses, all of which are linked to known malignancies.

82   D

Screening tests are becoming popular in the UK with most health strategies aimed at prevention and early detection as opposed to cure of disease. For a national screening programme to be valid, certain prerequisites must be fulfilled. These include disease and test criteria as follows:

Disease criteria:

- Common disease
- Important health problem
- Should have a long premorbid latent period
- Should be asymptomatic
- Should be detectable at an early stage
- Should be treatable by defined means in a cost-effective way at the time of detection

Test criteria:

- Highly sensitive and specific
- Non-invasive
- Must be able to be audited
- Cost-effective and acceptable to patients
- The test or its results should be without harm to the patient

Screening tests are not designed to detect early recurrence from primary disease.

83   B

Risk factors for breast cancer include female sex, older age, early menarche and late menopause, nulliparity, late first birth age, family history of breast cancer, atypical breast hyperplasia, and geographical location.

84   D

SIRS (systemic inflammatory response syndrome) is the syndrome resulting from the body's reaction to a critical illness. Defining criteria include:

Temperature >38°C or <36°C

Heart rate >90/min

Respiratory rate >20/min or pCO_2 <4.3 kPa (32 mmHg)

WBC >12,000 or <4000 or >10% immature forms.

85   D

A serum lactate level of >4 mmol/L is associated with a 50% mortality rate in any disease and should be taken very seriously. Haemorrhagic free fluid found at surgery indicates bowel infarction and should prompt a search for dead bowel with a view to resection. Atrial fibrillation, low oxygen saturation and high white cell counts are all indicators of systemic disease; however, if the original disease process is treated in addition to adequate oxygen and fluid resuscitation, then these parameters should resolve themselves.

86   A

There is still much debate about the use of early steroid therapy in the management of ARDS. Proven treatment strategies at present include, but are not limited to: prone position ventilation, activated protein C administration in sepsis, inverse ratio ventilation, inhaled nitric oxide use, management of the initial disease, nutritional support and early goal-directed therapy, mechanical ventilation with small tidal volumes and permissive hypercarbia, and strict control of fluid resuscitation.

87   D

To proceed with organ donation in a brainstem dead donor, the tests of brainstem death must be verified by two separate senior physicians after exclusion of endocrine, metabolic, therapeutic, and hypothermic abnormalities which may mask the examination. The test is in two sections, one to assess the lack of respiratory drive, and the second to establish brainstem inadequacy.

Lack of respiratory drive following hypercarbia:

The subject is pre-oxygenated with 100% oxygen and then disconnected from the ventilator for 10 minutes. The pCO_2 is allowed to rise and a level of >6.5 kPa should stimulate respiration in a normal but not brainstem dead individual.

Brainstem tests:

- Absent papillary and corneal reflexes
- Absent cranial nerve functioning
- Absent gag and cough reflexes
- Cold caloric test to demonstrate lack of vestibule-ocular reflexes.

Spinal reflexes are not relevant in brainstem death testing as they may very well be present in brain-dead individuals if the spinal cord has not sustained any injuries.

88   D

Massive blood transfusion is defined as a transfusion equivalent to the patient's blood volume administered within 24 hours. Complications of massive blood transfusion include volume overload, thrombocytopenia, coagulopathy, hypothermia, hypocalcaemia, and hyperkalaemia.
Hypocalcaemia occurs owing to the chelation of calcium by the citrate in the additive solution in stored blood.

89   E

Patients on steroids undergoing surgery require peri-operative steroid replacement in order to prevent an Addisonian crisis. This is dependent on the level of surgery and includes:

- **Minor surgery:** 50 mg IV hydrocortisone pre-operatively with continuation of oral steroids immediately after resuming oral intake.

- **Intermediate:** 50 mg hydrocortisone IV pre-operatively and 6-hourly for the first 24 hours and then switch to oral.

- **Major surgery:** 100 mg hydrocortisone IV pre-operatively and then 100 mg 6-hourly for at least the first 72 hours.

90   C

ASA 1 – normal healthy individual

ASA 2 – patient with mild systemic disease

ASA 3 – patient with severe systemic disease that limits activity but is not incapacitating

ASA 4 – incapacitating systemic disease that is constantly life-threatening

ASA 5 – moribund, not expected to survive 24 hours with or without surgery.

This patient has activity limiting severe systemic disease, but is not regarded as constantly life-threatening to be classed as ASA 4. Had this patient come in with an emergency condition, the acute problem may strain the pre-existing systemic diseases and lead to a reclassification as ASA 4.

PRACTICE PAPER 2: QUESTIONS

PRACTICE PAPER 2: QUESTIONS

1 **Which one of the following statements is correct regarding acoustic neuroma?**

○ A   acoustic neuromas make up 1% of all intracranial tumours

○ B   the majority are bilateral

○ C   vertigo is a common symptom

○ D   acoustic neuromas arise from Schwann cells

○ E   most patients have normal hearing

2 **Which of the following statements is TRUE about pharyngeal pouch?**

○ A   is also known as Zenker's diverticulum

○ B   arises from the anterior pharyngeal wall, known as Killian's dehiscence

○ C   hoarseness is a common symptom

○ D   barium swallow should not performed because of the risk of perforation

○ E   commonly, a pouch may contain an invasive squamous cell carcinoma (SCC) in its wall

3   Which of the following is the commonest cause of vocal cord palsy in an adult?

○ A   idiopathic

○ B   malignant disease

○ C   trauma

○ D   cerebrovascular accidents

○ E   iatrogenic

4   A 1st year medical student attends a dental appointment for a filling of a right lower 7th molar tooth under local anaesthetic. After injection of the anaesthetic, she notices that her right half of the chin has gone numb; however, she still retains normal movements of the jaw. Which of the following nerves has been infiltrated by local anaesthetic in this clinical scenario?

○ A   lingual nerve

○ B   buccal nerve

○ C   mental nerve

○ D   mandibular nerve

○ E   inferior alveolar nerve

5   Which of the following structures are skeletal derivatives of the 3rd branchial arch?

○ A   stapes

○ B   styloid process

○ C   incus and malleus

○ D   lesser cornu of the hyoid bone

○ E   greater cornu of the hyoid bone

6   All of the following sinuses drain into the middle meatus below the middle concha of the maxilla EXCEPT the

⚪   A   posterior ethmoidal sinus

⚪   B   middle ethmoidal sinus

⚪   C   anterior ethmoidal sinus

⚪   D   frontal sinus

⚪   E   maxillary sinus

7   A 4-year-old child is brought into the Emergency Department by his mother after having fallen from a slide at a height of 2 metres. His vitals are HR 135/min, BP 90/70, respiratory rate 28/min, and temperature 36.5°C. Which one of the following signs would you consider abnormal in this child?

⚪   A   heart rate

⚪   B   blood pressure

⚪   C   respiratory rate

⚪   D   temperature

⚪   E   none of the above

8   Children born with Down syndrome (trisomy 21) are associated with an increased risk of all of the following surgical conditions EXCEPT

⚪   A   endocardial cushion defect

⚪   B   cryptorchidism

⚪   C   duodenal atresia

⚪   D   diaphragmatic hernia

⚪   E   Hirschsprung's disease

9   All of the following features are associated with necrotising enterocolitis EXCEPT

○ A   pneumatosis coli

○ B   bleeding per rectum

○ C   metabolic acidosis

○ D   haematemesis

○ E   disseminated intravascular coagulation

10   A complete division of the right oculomotor nerve (III) would result in all of the following signs EXCEPT

○ A   ptosis

○ B   diplopia

○ C   convergent squint

○ D   dilated pupil on the right side

○ E   loss of a consensual pupillary reflex when the left eye is examined

11   A 66-year-old male comes into the Emergency Department with severe tearing chest pain, which radiates to the back. His past medical history includes hypertension and diet-controlled diabetes. Examination reveals an early diastolic murmur and blood pressure differences in both arms of >15 mmHg. The gold standard investigation of choice in confirming your diagnosis would be

○ A   CT chest with contrast

○ B   MRI chest

○ C   echocardiogram

○ D   electrocardiogram

○ E   angiogram of the arch vessels

12 Which of the following vessels used in coronary artery bypass grafting, has been shown through evidence-based practice to have the best outcome for long-term graft patency rates?

- ⬭ A   internal thoracic artery
- ⬭ B   radial artery
- ⬭ C   long saphenous vein
- ⬭ D   short saphenous vein
- ⬭ E   cephalic vein

13 Which of the following diseases is the commonest indication for a bilateral lung transplant?

- ⬭ A   chronic obstructive pulmonary disease
- ⬭ B   primary pulmonary hypertension
- ⬭ C   fibrotic lung disease
- ⬭ D   cystic fibrosis
- ⬭ E   severe asbestosis

14 Which of the following statements regarding dumping syndrome is correct?

- ⬭ A   may be avoided by performing a gastroenterostomy
- ⬭ B   results from hyperosmolar fluid reaching the small bowel
- ⬭ C   is reduced by eating high carbohydrate meals frequently
- ⬭ D   may cause constipatory symptoms
- ⬭ E   may be avoided by pylorus-preserving surgery

15 All of the following staements about a hiatus hernia are correct EXCEPT

- ○ A   they are more common in males
- ○ B   rolling types are more common than sliding
- ○ C   sliding types are more common in the elderly
- ○ D   dysphagia is accounted for by extrinsic compression
- ○ E   gastric volvulus is rare

16 Which of the following cases should be considered to have the highest priority on the emergency theatre list?

- ○ A   laparoscopic appendicectomy for suspected appendicitis
- ○ B   pyloroplasty for congenital pyloric stenosis
- ○ C   incarcerated inguinal hernia in a young man
- ○ D   strangulated femoral hernia in an elderly woman
- ○ E   hemiarthroplasty for fractured neck of femur

17 Which of the following hepatobiliary conditions would typically result in an unconjugated hyperbilirubinaemia?

- ○ A   Crigler–Najjar syndrome
- ○ B   primary biliary cirrhosis
- ○ C   Mirrizi syndrome
- ○ D   congenital biliary atresia
- ○ E   hepatitis B infection

18 The following are all recognised complications of acute pancreatitis EXCEPT

- ○ A toxic psychosis
- ○ B gastric ulceration
- ○ C chronic renal failure
- ○ D pancreatic abscess
- ○ E hypocalcaemia

19 A 34-year-old woman undergoes a right mastectomy and axillary clearance for a 4 cm carcinoma of the right breast with fixed unilateral axillary nodes. A staging CT scan confirms that there are no metastases present. Which of the following TNM stages does this patient's clinical picture represent?

- ○ A T1 N0 M0
- ○ B T1 N1 M0
- ○ C T2 N0 M0
- ○ D T2 N1 M0
- ○ E T2 N2 M0

20 A 42-year-old woman attends your clinic to discuss her management options following her results of a triple assessment scan. She is found to have ductal carcinoma in-situ (DCIS) on Tru-cut biopsy of a 5 cm mass in her right breast. Which of the following treatment options would you advise for this woman?

- A right mastectomy
- B right mastectomy with axillary clearance
- C right mastectomy with sentinel node biopsy
- D right wide local excision
- E right wide local excision with axillary clearance

21 A 24-year-old woman, who is 2 months' post-partum and is breastfeeding, attends your clinic with symptomatic hyperthyroidism. Which of the following treatments would you initiate in this patient to treat her hyperthyroidism?

- A radioactive iodine
- B carbimazole
- C proplythiouracil
- D atenolol therapy
- E iodine therapy with recommended cessation of breastfeeding

22   A 35-year-old woman presents to your endocrine clinic with complaints of lethargy and easy skin bruising. She appears to have cushingoid features and you decide to investigate this in the outpatients' department with some simple blood tests. All of the following are features of Cushing's disease found on blood testing EXCEPT

- ○ A   hypernatraemia
- ○ B   hypokalaemia
- ○ C   hyperglycaemia
- ○ D   lowered plasma adrenocorticotropic hormone (ACTH)
- ○ E   raised plasma cortisol levels

23   The commonest site for peripheral vascular aneurysms after the aorta is

- ○ A   iliac artery
- ○ B   femoral artery
- ○ C   popliteal artery
- ○ D   splenic artery
- ○ E   radial artery

24   Which of the following statements is true?

○   A   veins are better than arteries as conduits for bypass procedures

○   B   superficial veins may be stripped in the presence of deep venous insufficiency

○   C   the radial artery is safe to be harvested if Allen's test reveals a time of 15 seconds

○   D   veins may need valves to be stripped with a valvulotome before use in bypass procedures

○   E   off-pump coronary artery bypass graft (CABG) procedures increase the risk of transient ischaemic attack (TIA) or cerebrovascular accident (CVA)

25   Which of the following ulcers are correctly associated?

○   A   Cushing's ulcer – burns

○   B   venous ulcer – haemochromatosis

○   C   Curling's ulcer – head injury

○   D   neuropathic ulcer – glucosuria

○   E   Marjolin's ulcer – chronic scarring

26   In acute arterial occlusion, the tissue that is most sensitive to arterial hypoxaemia is

○   A   skin

○   B   subcutaneous tissue

○   C   nerve

○   D   muscle

○   E   bone

27 A 34-year-old male wants to donate a kidney to his sister. His BMI is 31. His GFR is 110 mL/min. The patient and his sister have the same blood group but they have no HLA antigens in common. On arteriography, he has a single renal artery and single renal vein on the left and single renal artery and single vein on the right. Based on the above findings which of the following statements is true?

○ A the patient and his sister do not have the same biological parents

○ B the patient is too overweight to be a living kidney donor

○ C the patient's kidney function is not adequate for him to be a donor

○ D the kidney of choice for donation and transplant is the left kidney

○ E the kidney of choice for donation and transplant is the right kidney

28 A 25-year-old right-handed young woman is brought into the Emergency Department after a traumatic amputation of her right middle finger less than 1 hour ago. The finger has been preserved on ice and a decision is taken to re-implant the finger under general anaesthetic. The correct order in which the structures will be re-anastomosed (excluding the finger tendons) includes which of the following?

○ A artery, vein, bone, nerve, skin

○ B artery, bone, vein, nerve, skin

○ C bone, artery, vein, nerve, skin

○ D bone, vein, artery, nerve, skin

○ E vein, artery, bone, nerve, skin

29 A 45-year-old patient presents to Casualty one hour after falling
from his mountain bike. He is complaining of left hip pain and
X-rays reveal an undisplaced intracapsular fracture of his left
femoral neck. The best method of treatment for this patient is

○ A   dynamic hip screw

○ B   hemiarthroplasty

○ C   partially threaded cancellous screws

○ D   intramedullary reconstruction nail

○ E   total hip replacement

30 A 50-year-old female has a Colles' fracture manipulated in theatre,
followed by application of a full below elbow cast. One hour after
being on the ward with her arm elevated, she starts to complain of
paraesthaesia in the index and middle fingers along with wrist
pain. The correct initial treatment should be

○ A   observe for another hour to see if the symptoms settle

○ B   split the cast and lower the arm

○ C   take her back to theatre for a remanipulation

○ D   split the cast and keep the arm elevated

○ E   perform an urgent carpal tunnel decompression

31   The conjoint tendon of the biceps and coracobrachialis is
retracted medially during an anterior approach to the shoulder.
Postoperatively the patient has weakness of elbow flexion and
reduced sensation over the lateral forearm. Which nerve has been
clinically injured?

○   A   radial

○   B   median

○   C   ulnar

○   D   musculocutaneous

○   E   axillary

32   In the spine, the intervertebral disc, which is most commonly
implicated for causing nerve root symptoms, is the disc between

○   A   L5/S1

○   B   L4/5

○   C   L3/4

○   D   L1/2

○   E   T12/L1

33 **All of the following statements about carcinoma of the gallbladder are correct EXCEPT**

○ A   the neoplasm usually starts in the cystic duct and neck of the gallbladder

○ B   it is found more commonly in women than men

○ C   it is associated with the presence of gallstones in >85% of cases

○ D   prognosis is generally poor with <1 year survival with local invasion

○ E   chemotherapy and radiotherapy do not alter disease progression

34 **All of the following statements about herceptin are correct EXCEPT**

○ A   it is a form of immunotherapy as opposed to chemotherapy

○ B   patients receiving herceptin need regular cardiac function monitoring

○ C   it can be used in combination with paclitaxel as a first-line agent for metastatic breast cancer with HER–2 overexpression

○ D   up to 40% of patients may get an infusion reaction in the first 24 hours

○ E   polycythaemia and leukaemia may occur

35 Which of the following statements regarding malignant bone tumours is correct?

- ○ A primary malignant bone tumours account for 3% of all deaths from malignant disease in the UK

- ○ B Ewing's sarcoma is more common in prevalence than chondrosarcoma

- ○ C pain is an unusual presenting feature of bone tumours

- ○ D the commonest presenting site of an osteosarcoma is the proximal femur and proximal humerus

- ○ E radiographic features of an osteosarcoma reveal a sclerotic intramedullary lesion of the metaphysis

36 Following pneumonectomy for carcinoma of the lung, which of the following statement is true?

- ○ A a chest drain is always required

- ○ B mortality rates are higher for left-sided pneumonectomy compared to right side

- ○ C bronchopleural fistulae occur in <5% of cases

- ○ D a double-lumen endotracheal tube is contraindicated

- ○ E mediastinal shift is a major problem requiring further surgery

37 A 23-year-old male is brought into the A&E department after having been involved in a motorbike accident at high speeds. He is unconscious and has a cervical collar on as a C-spine injury cannot be excluded without X-rays. A decision to intubate him using the nasotracheal route is taken. Contraindications to blind nasotracheal intubation in this patient would include all of the following EXCEPT

○ A   apnoea

○ B   cervical spine injury

○ C   skull base fracture

○ D   frontal bone fracture

○ E   facial fractures

38 Complications of a surgical cricothyroidotomy include all of the following EXCEPT

○ A   subglottic stenosis

○ B   mediastinal emphysema

○ C   vocal cord paralysis

○ D   oesophageal laceration

○ E   carotid artery puncture

39 A 24-year-old male is brought into the A&E department having sustained multiple stab wound injuries to the chest and abdomen. His HR is 130/min, BP 90/50, RR 34/min, with a narrow pulse pressure and reduced urine output. Given this clinical scenario, how much blood volume loss do you expect in this patient?

- ○ A 600 mL
- ○ B 950 mL
- ○ C 1300 mL
- ○ D 1650 mL
- ○ E 2000 mL

40 How much crystalloid fluid volume resuscitation does this patient require immediately as cross-matched blood is being awaited?

- ○ A 1900 mL
- ○ B 2600 mL
- ○ C 3300 mL
- ○ D 3900 mL
- ○ E 4950 mL

41 A 60-year-old male smoker who is under your care undergoes a laryngectomy for cancer of the larynx. In assessing the sterility of this operation, you would best classify this procedure as a

- ○ A clean procedure
- ○ B clean-contaminated procedure
- ○ C contaminated procedure
- ○ D contaminated-dirty procedure
- ○ E dirty procedure

42   An advantage of using povidone-iodine disinfectant over chlorhexidine solution while a surgical scrub is being performed is that iodine

- A   causes less skin sensitivity and irritation than does chlorhexidine
- B   has a longer duration of action than chlorhexidine
- C   is more effective than chlorhexidine against spores and fungi
- D   has greater bactericidal activity than chlorhexidine for Gram-positive bacteria
- E   is resistant to deactivation in the presence of organic material such as blood, pus and faeces

43   A 14-year-old girl is admitted as an in-patient under your care with suspected acute appendicitis. She is competent to understand the diagnosis and management decision along with complications of undergoing an appendicectomy. She consents to the procedure; however, her parents do not want her to undergo the treatment as your diagnosis is not guaranteed, and fear that their daughter may undergo unnecessary surgery.
Assuming that this case has been discussed with all relevant hospital personnel and team members, which of the following options should you carry on with?

- A   proceed against the parents' wishes to an appendicetomy
- B   agree with the parents' wishes and withhold from operating
- C   obtain a court order to carry out treatment in the patient's best interests
- D   adopt a 'wait and see' policy in this particular case
- E   treat the patient with antibiotics in the first instance

44 **Which of the following statements regarding monopolar diathermy is true?**

○ A   it uses a very high frequency direct current to cut and coagulate

○ B   cutting of tissues is accomplished by pulsed output of currents at short intervals

○ C   currents as high as 500 mA can be passed through the body at frequencies of 5 mHz

○ D   when monopolar diathermy forceps are used, the current is passed between the two limbs of the forceps at the tip

○ E   it can be used in surgery on the penis or digits

45 **Capacitance coupling in laparoscopic surgery can be avoided by**

○ A   careful use of prep solution

○ B   having the surgery performed by the most experienced surgeon available

○ C   use of an insulated instrument with a metal cannula

○ D   use of all metal instruments and cannula

○ E   use of lower power settings on the diathermy machine

46 **All of the following special precautions should be taken when operating on a patient with known HIV status EXCEPT**

○ A   use of disposable gowns and drapes

○ B   double gloving and use of indicator systems

○ C   minimising the presence of unnecessary theatre staff

○ D   operating in a theatre with negative pressure air ventilation

○ E   use of the kidney dish to pass all instruments

47   All of the following statements regarding the anion gap are true
EXCEPT

○   A   normal range is between 10 and 19 mmol/L

○   B   it reflects the concentrations of normally unmeasured anions in
the serum

○   C   it will be abnormal in conditions where bicarbonate is lost such
as diarrhoea and fistulae

○   D   it is calculated by taking the difference between the main cations
and anions in the serum (Na, K, HCO_3, Cl)

○   E   it would be increased in the serum of a runner immediately after
a marathon

48   You are looking after a 73-year-old woman in ITU who requires
total parenteral nutrition (TPN) via a central venous catheter in
her right internal jugular vein. All of the following are recognised
complications of central venous pressure (CVP) line insertion
EXCEPT

○   A   tension pneumothorax

○   B   air embolus

○   C   cardiac arrythmias

○   D   pleural effusions

○   E   thrombophlebitis

49   **Which of the following statements about immediate care of a patient with burns is correct?**

○   A   third degree burns are usually painless

○   B   IV lines may be placed in burnt skin provided no other site is accessible and good venous access is obtained

○   C   priority is given to the airway and breathing before attending to stop the burning process

○   D   fluid resuscitation is calculated by a formula involving the body weight, percentage area burned, and the degree of burns

○   E   the most important complication found in the hospital phase of recovery from a large (>40%) burn is renal failure

50   **All of the following signs are found in refeeding syndrome EXCEPT**

○   A   hypophosphataemia

○   B   hypocalcaemia

○   C   hypokalaemia

○   D   hypoglycaemia

○   E   hypomagnesaemia

51–53   For the following questions regarding blood gas interpretations, please select from the one of the following best answers. Each clinical scenario has one best answer. Each answer may be used more than once or not at all

- [ ]   A   uncompensated metabolic acidosis
- [ ]   B   uncompensated respiratory acidosis
- [ ]   C   compensated metabolic acidosis
- [ ]   D   compensated respiratory acidosis
- [ ]   E   mixed metabolic acidosis with metabolic alkalosis

51   A 23-year-old female patient has just been admitted following an aspirin overdose. She does not state how many tablets she has ingested; however, she is complaining of tinnitus. She has vomited six times before presenting and appears to be tachypnoeic on arrival to the A&E. Her blood gas reveals the following: pH 7.4; HCO_3 22; BE –2; pCO_2 5 kPa

52   You are asked to review a patient who is 2 days post-laparotomy for a perforated duodenal ulcer. On blood gases, the following results are noted: pH 7.35; HCO_3 35; BE +9; pCO_2 7 kPa

53   A 33-year-old insulin-dependent diabetic patient attends the day surgery unit for an inguinal hernia repair on the afternoon list. In the anaesthetic room, she collapses and is immediately resuscitated by the anaesthetist present. A blood gas taken shows pH 7.2; HCO_3 12; BE –14; pCO_2 5.3 kPa

54 Which of the following pathological changes are correctly associated with the named diseases?

○ A   familial adenomatous polyp (FAP) – metaplasia

○ B   Peutz–Jehger's – hamartoma

○ C   Barratt's oesophagus – dysplasia

○ D   Paget's disease of the nipple – metaplasia

○ E   Gardner's syndrome – hamartoma

55 Presence of all of the following factors will predispose to the development of an anal fistula EXCEPT

○ A   infection

○ B   foreign bodies

○ C   radiation

○ D   neoplastic disease

○ E   inadequate vascularisation

56 Which of the following statements regarding FAP is true?

○ A   it accounts for up to 10% of colorectal carcinomas

○ B   it may be treated with a prophylactic right hemicolectomy

○ C   it usually takes 30–40 years to present as a colorectal carcinoma

○ D   the gene is located on the long arm of chromosome 5

○ E   it is inherited as autosomal recessive

57   **Which of the following statements is correct regarding complement function?**

O   A   C5a – cytolytic activity

O   B   C3a – neutrophil chemotaxis

O   C   C3b – release of histamine from mast cells

O   D   C8 – neutrophil chemotaxis

O   E   C7 – cytolytic activity

58   **All of the following familial cancer syndromes are correctly associated with the resultant neoplasm EXCEPT**

O   A   Li–Fraumeni – cerebral astrocytomas

O   B   retinoblastoma (Rb1) – osteosarcomas

O   C   Von Hipple–Lindau (VHL) – renal carcinoma

O   D   BRCA1 and 2 – ovarian carcinoma

O   E   MEN 1 – phaeochromocytoma

59   **Which of the following statements regarding the spleen is correct?**

O   A   red pulp consists of central arteries ensheathed by lymphoid nodules and lymphocytes

O   B   red pulp forms most of the splenic volume

O   C   most of the antibody synthesis in the spleen occurs in the red pulp

O   D   white pulp contains sinusoids, which trap defective red cells

O   E   white pulp contains B lymphocytes located immediately in the vicinity of the central artery

60 Which of the following phases in a cell cycle is the most resistant to chemotherapeutic agents and requires higher doses in order to obtain a response?

○ A G_0

○ B G_1

○ C   S

○ D G_2

○ E   M

61 A 55-year-old man on the surgical high dependency unit is being treated with dobutamine for congestive heart failure. The mechanism of action of dobutamine is

○ A α-adrenergic agonist

○ B β-adrenergic agonist

○ C β-cholinergic agonist

○ D α- and β-cholinergic agonist

○ E α- and β-adrenergic agonist

62 **All of the following mechanisms are involved in the secretion of gastric acid EXCEPT**

- ○ A release of ACh from the vagus nerve in response to gastric distension
- ○ B release of gastrin from the G-cells in response to acetylcholine stimulation
- ○ C release of gastrin from the G-cells in response to histamine stimulation
- ○ D release of histamine from the enterochromaffin cells to act on the parietal cells
- ○ E neural stimulation arising from the hypothalamus in anticipation of food ingestion

63 **All of the following vitamins are synthesised in the gut by colonic bacteria EXCEPT**

- ○ A vitamin K
- ○ B vitamin B_{12}
- ○ C vitamin B_2 (riboflavin)
- ○ D vitamin B_1 (thiamine)
- ○ E vitamin B_3 (niacin)

64   The main effect of ADH (antidiuretic hormone) on the kidney is to

○   A   reduce urine volume production by decreasing the GFR

○   B   concentrate the urine by increasing Na^+ excretion

○   C   increase water retention by upregulating Na/K receptors in the distal nephron

○   D   increase water retention by increasing distal nephron permeability to water

○   E   increase water retention by increasing Na^+ resorption by acting on the Na/K ATPase pump in the distal nephron

65   Which one of the following associations of daily GI secretion volume (in a normal 70 kg young adult) and fluid type are correctly associated?

○   A   saliva – 0.5 L

○   B   gastric juice – 2 L

○   C   bile – 0.2 L

○   D   pancreatic juice – 3 L

○   E   intestinal secretions – 5 L

66   All of the following conditions would result in decreased lung compliance EXCEPT

○   A α_1-antitrypsin deficiency

○   B   pulmonary oedema

○   C   supine position

○   D   mechanical ventilation

○   E   increased age

67   Regarding pulmonary blood flow, which of the following statements is correct?

○   A   both hypoxia and hypercapnia result in constriction of smaller alveolar vessels

○   B   hypercapnia results in dilatation of smaller alveolar vessels

○   C   pulmonary arterioles play an important role in the regulation of pulmonary blood flow

○   D   perfusion of blood with alveolar ventilation is better matched towards the base of the lung rather than the apex

○   E   perfusion of blood with alveolar ventilation is better matched towards the apex of the lung rather than the base

68   Which of the following statements is true regarding HbF (fetal haemoglobin)?

○   A   HbF contains 2α and 2β chains in its structure

○   B   the oxygen dissociation curve for HbF is shifted to the left because of the decreased affinity for O_2

○   C   HbF responds to an increase in 2,3-DPG by a right shift towards the adult Hb curve

○   D   HbF production is increased with the administration of erythropoietin (Epo)

○   E   decreased levels are found in patients from African and Arabian populations

69   Which of the following statements regarding ANP (atrial naturetic peptide) is correct?

○   A   it stimulates ADH secretion

○   B   it increases the GFR by simultaneous dilatation of renal afferent arterioles and constriction of efferent arterioles

○   C   it is secreted in response to hyponatraemia

○   D   secretion increases as central venous pressure decreases

○   E   it acts on selected parts of the nephron to increase water and salt resorption

70   A 43-year-old postman presents to your clinic with troublesome PR bleeding and feeling of a prolapse. Examination reveals 3rd degree haemorrhoids. Ideal management of this patient would include which of the following treatment options?

○   A   injection sclerotherapy

○   B   banding of piles

○   C   prolapse and haemorrhoidopexy (PPH)

○   D   open haemorrhoidectomy with a Delorme's procedure for prolapse

○   E   fibre diet alone and observe in the outpatient setting

71   **Which of the following statements is true regarding the aetiology of colorectal carcinoma?**

○   A   Crohn's disease poses a similar risk in the development of colorectal carcinoma as does ulcerative colitis

○   B   malignancy developing from ureterosigmoidostomy classically occurs at some distance from the anastomosis site

○   C   colon cancer is more prevalent in non-urban areas compared with urban

○   D   HNPCC causes over 60% of tumours proximal to the splenic flexure

○   E   Gardner's syndrome results from a mutation on chromosome 6

72   **Which of the following statements are true regarding the management of colorectal carcinoma?**

○   A   5-FU is commonly used in the adjuvant treatment of Duke's B colon cancer

○   B   postoperative adjuvant radiotherapy for locally extensive but resectable colon cancer is preferred over pre-operative radiation

○   C   patients presenting with large bowel obstruction from an ascending colon tumour are best treated with a primary resection with a defunctioning colostomy to aid healing of the anastomosis

○   D   surveillance colonoscopy should be performed annually for the first 10 years to assess the presence of local recurrence and metachronous tumours

○   E   hand-sewn anastomoses in bowel resections for cancer have been shown to be structurally and functionally superior to stapled anastomosis

73 **All of the following are true statements regarding diverticular disease EXCEPT**

○ A it is found more commonly in the developed world

○ B surgical treatment is usually unnecessary in acute uncomplicated disease

○ C diverticulae are most commonly found in the descending colon

○ D perforation and fistula formation can result from an attack of acute diverticulitis

○ E resolution of the diverticulae can occur with high fibre diets and adequate hydration

74 **A 54-year-old woman in-patient is referred to your surgical team with a diagnosis of small bowel obstruction. Which one of the following clinical signs would you look for in trying to identify the commonest cause of this condition?**

○ A previous abdominal surgery scar

○ B lump in the groin above and medial to the pubic tubercle

○ C lump in the groin below and lateral to the pubic tubercle

○ D cachexia and nodule at the umbilicus

○ E circumoral pigmentation and a family history of previous obstruction

75 All of the following causes of peptic ulceration may be cured by a course of proton pump inhibitor (PPI) therapy EXCEPT

- ○ A non-steroidal anti-inflammatory drug (NSAID)-induced ulceration
- ○ B *Helicobacter pylori* ulceration in addition to triple therapy
- ○ C Cushing's ulceration
- ○ D Curling's ulceration
- ○ E Zollinger–Ellison syndrome

76 All of the following statements regarding renal artery stenosis are true EXCEPT

- ○ A it can cause acute renal failure in patients who are taking ACE inhibitor therapy
- ○ B it is a cause of secondary hypertension
- ○ C it is most commonly caused by atherosclerosis in younger patients
- ○ D treatment may include stenting of the involved vessels
- ○ E it may lead to hypokalaemia

77 A 14-year-old boy is referred from A&E to you with sudden onset right-sided testicular pain of 6 hours' duration. On examination, you find the right testicle is hard, swollen, and lying transversely with severe tenderness on light palpation. The next step in management is

- ○ A urgent ultrasound scan of the testis
- ○ B analgesia, antibiotics and outpatient follow-up
- ○ C urgent theatre for testicular exploration
- ○ D admission for observation and analgesia
- ○ E elective arrangement for bilateral orchidoplexy

78 The following are all management options in the definitive treatment of urethral strictures EXCEPT

- ○ A optical urethrotomy
- ○ B open urethroplasty
- ○ C urethral dilators
- ○ D urethral catheterisation
- ○ E urethral stenting

79 All of the following are correct boundaries of the foramen of Winslow EXCEPT

- ○ A free edge of the lesser omentum
- ○ B inferior vena cava posteriorly
- ○ C first part of the duodenum
- ○ D quadrate lobe of the liver
- ○ E porta hepatis

80 The following layers of tissue are encountered during a Pfannensteil incision EXCEPT

- ○ A subcutaneous tissue layers of camper and scarpa
- ○ B anterior rectus sheath
- ○ C linea alba
- ○ D posterior rectus sheath
- ○ E peritoneum

81   A 55-year-old woman is referred to you by the GP with an adenocarcinoma of the distal transverse colon recently found on colonoscopy and biopsy. Following the MDT meeting, a decision to undertake an extended right hemicolectomy is agreed. You realise that all of the following structures may be at risk of damage from direct or indirect effects when extended right hemicolectomy is performed EXCEPT

○ A   right ureter

○ B   right gonadal vessels

○ C   fourth part of the duodenum

○ D   right ovary or testis

○ E   spleen

82   Whilst performing a small bowel resection for strictures following Crohn's disease, you realise that on inspection, there are marked differences between jejunal and ileal anatomy. Such differences include all of the following EXCEPT

○ A   wider lumen in the jejunum

○ B   less lymphatics in the jejunal mesentery compared to ileal

○ C   more prominent and multiple arcades of vessels in the ileum

○ D   thicker wall of the ileum

○ E   thicker and more fat-laden mesentery increasing towards the ileum

83   A 67-year-old man who is an in-patient on your ward undergoes a
      thyroidectomy and right radical neck dissection. On the first post-
      operative day he complains that he is unable to initiate shoulder
      abduction. Which one of the following nerves is most likely to be
      injured?

      ○   A   axillary nerve
      ○   B   suprascapular nerve
      ○   C   dorsal scapular nerve
      ○   D   lateral pectoral nerve
      ○   E   thoracodorsal nerve

84   A 23-year-old male sustains a stab wound to his cubital fossa
      during a fight. You suspect that there may be damage to the
      median nerve. All of the following muscles would lose their motor
      innervation EXCEPT

      ○   A   palmaris longus
      ○   B   abductor pollicis brevis
      ○   C   pronator teres
      ○   D   adductor pollicis
      ○   E   opponens pollicis

85   All of the following arteries are named direct branches of the
      axillary artery EXCEPT

      ○   A   superior thoracic artery
      ○   B   lateral thoracic artery
      ○   C   suprascapular artery
      ○   D   subscapular artery
      ○   E   acromiothoracic artery

86   The following are true statements about the trachea EXCEPT

- A   the trachea commences at the cricoid cartilage at C6
- B   the trachea ends at the bifurcation (carina) at the level of the 2nd rib
- C   the tracheal bifurcation varies with respiration between T4 and T6
- D   the trachea is laterally related to the thyroid lobes and carotid arteries
- E   the trachea is lined by stratified squamous non-keratinising epithelium

87   A 65-year-old male ex-smoker undergoes a single left main-stem LIMA coronary artery bypass grafting operation by a median sternotomy approach. During the recovery period 1 week post-operatively, it is noted that he still has a persistent hoarse voice after extubation 5 days earlier. The nerve most likely to be damaged during surgery is

- A   right recurrent laryngeal nerve
- B   superior laryngeal nerve
- C   left recurrent laryngeal nerve
- D   left phrenic nerve
- E   right phrenic nerve

88 All of the following muscles are lateral rotators of the hip joint EXCEPT

- ○ A gluteus maximus
- ○ B pectineus
- ○ C gemellus superior
- ○ D obturator externus
- ○ E quadratus femoris

89 A 16-year-old boy is brought into the Emergency Department after having injured his right knee during a rugby game. After careful history-taking, the injury he describes indicates that his knee was forcibly abducted and externally rotated whilst in a flexed position. This scenario would classically result in a tear of

- ○ A anterior cruciate ligament
- ○ B posterior cruciate ligament
- ○ C medial meniscus
- ○ D lateral meniscus
- ○ E lateral collateral ligament

90 Structures passing through the greater sciatic foramen include all of the following EXCEPT

- ○ A piriformis muscle
- ○ B posterior cutaneous nerve of the thigh
- ○ C nerve to obturator internus
- ○ D tendon of obturator internus
- ○ E internal pudendal artery

PRACTICE PAPER 2: ANSWERS AND TEACHING NOTES

PRACTICE PAPER 2: ANSWERS AND TEACHING NOTES

1   D

Acoustic neuromas arise from Schwann cells and make up 8% of all intracranial tumours. The majority are unilateral (95%). Patients usually present with gradual progressive unilateral deafness (90%) associated with tinnitus (70%). Vertigo is unusual. The investigation of choice is a gadolinium-enhanced MRI scan.

2   A

Pharyngeal pouches arise from Killian's dehiscence, which is a posterior pharyngeal weakness between thyropharyngeus and cricopharyngeus. It is also known as Zenker's diverticulum. Patients may present with a lump in the throat, dysphagia and regurgitation of food. Only very rarely may a pouch contain an invasive SCC. Barium swallow is the initial definitive investigation.

3   B

Unilateral vocal cord palsy produces hoarseness. The commonest cause is malignant disease (30%), especially of the bronchus followed by iatrogenic causes (25%), ie thyroid surgery or any surgery along the course of the recurrent laryngeal nerve. Trauma, idiopathic and other causes, eg central and myopathies, are unlikely (15% each).

4   E

The branches of the posterior division of the mandibular nerve supply the tongue and oral cavity. The lingual nerve is sensory to the anterior two-thirds of the tongue and also contains within it the chorda tympani branch, which allows for detection of taste. The inferior alveolar nerve branch passes through the inferior alveolar foramen of the mandible and supplies sensation to the lower teeth. This nerve ends as the mental nerve as it emerges from the mental foramen to supply sensation to the skin overlying the chin and lower lip.

5   E

Skeletal derivatives of the 3rd branchial arch or 'thyrohyoid arch' include the inferior body and greater cornu of the hyoid bone. The remainder of the hyoid bone including the styloid process and stapes are derived from the 2nd brachial arch or 'hyoid arch'. The incus and malleus are derivatives of the 1st branchial arch.

6   A

The posterior ethmoidal sinus drains into the superior recess underlying the superior concha. The remaining named sinuses drain below the middle concha.

7   E

Age (years)	HR (bpm)	BP (mmHg)	Resp rate (breaths/min)
0–1	<160	>60	<60
1–3	<150	>70	<40
3–5	<140	>75	<35
6–12	<120	>80	<30
>12	<100	>90	<30

8   D

Although case reports show that diaphragmatic hernias can occur in children with Down syndrome, there is no increased risk above that of the normal population. Endocardial cushion defects, duodenal atresia, Hirschsprung's disease, and cryptorchidism are all known associations with Down syndrome.

9   D

Necrotising enterocolitis (NEC) is the most common gastrointestinal surgical emergency occurring in neonates. With mortality rates approaching 50% in infants who weigh <1500 g, NEC represents a significant clinical problem.

Initial symptoms can include the following:

- feeding intolerance and delayed gastric emptying
- abdominal distention and/or tenderness
- hematochezia

Systemic signs can include the following:

- apnoea
- lethargy
- decreased peripheral perfusion and shock (in advanced stages)
- cardiovascular collapse
- bleeding diathesis (DIC)
- pneumatosis coli and metabolic acidosis result; however, haematemesis is not classically found in this condition.

10   C

All of the following signs are seen as well as a divergent squint. This occurs owing to the unopposed action of the lateral rectus and superior oblique muscles.

11   E

The gold standard in investigations for aortic dissection in a stable patient is an arch aortogram to assess accurately the extent and nature of the dissection. This is also essential in planning a surgical approach to treatment.

12   A

The internal thoracic or internal mammary artery has been demonstrated to have the best patency rates in the surgical treatment of coronary main vessel disease. The other vessels listed may be used. However, the long-term patency rates are not as great.

13   D

The only absolute indication for a bilateral lung transplant is cystic fibrosis. Other indications such as severe COPD, fibrosis and pulmonary hypertension are relative indications and may also be considered for single lung transplantation in certain cases.

14   B

Dumping syndrome occurs after gastrectomy surgery owing to the rapid emptying of hyperosmolar contents into the small bowel and causing a rapid fluid shift into the lumen of the bowel. Patients complain of dizziness, faintness, nausea, and vomiting within 15 minutes of eating a meal. Patients are advised to take small meals frequently with a low carbohydrate and high fibre component. A late dumping syndrome may result in a reactive hypoglycaemia from a delayed insulin secretory response.

15   C

Hiatus herniae are protrusions of viscus through the oesophageal hiatus. They are more common in the elderly and are usually (80%) of the sliding variety. Dysphagia is only reported in about 20% of patients and the most common symptom is upper abdominal discomfort.

16   D

A laparoscopic appendicectomy for suspected appendicitis should be done within 12 hours of diagnosis, although ideally as soon as possible. Patients may be maintained on IV antibiotics in the meanwhile. The laparoscopic approach should have no difference in priority from the open approach. Pyloroplasty for congenital pyloric stenosis should also be surgically operated within a day; however, neonates usually require a period of resuscitation pre-operatively due to the loss of fluid and electrolytes from all the vomiting. An incarcerated inguinal hernia in a young man that is not strangulated or obstructed can wait until the next elective list, provided it is not symptomatic. A strangulated femoral hernia in an elderly woman may contain ischaemic bowel and requires urgent operation. A long period of resuscitation is not recommended as the cause of any sepsis may worsen in delaying surgery. Hemiarthroplasty for fractured neck of the femur can wait at least a day before being booked onto the trauma list for surgery.

17   A

Unconjugated hyperbilirubinaemia results from prehepatic haemolysis or hepatic disorders of bilirubin conjugation such as Gilbert's syndrome and Crigler–Najjar syndrome. The remainder of causes listed result in jaundice from an elevated level of conjugated bilirubin.

18   C

Acute pancreatitis may cause acute renal failure, ARDS, and DIC in very severe cases. However, chronic (long-term) renal failure is not a recognised complication.

19   E

Tis – in-situ carcinoma
T1 – <2 cm
T2 – 2–5 cm
T3 – >5 cm
T4 – involvement of chest wall or skin

M0 – no distant metastases
M1 – distant metastases

N0 – No regional nodes
N1 – palpable unilateral axillary nodes
N2 – fixed unilateral axillary nodes
N3 – unilateral internal mammary nodes

20   C

A right mastectomy is recommended for any solid tumour >4 cm; however, this may also be dependent on general breast size, in which case, breast conserving surgery may be considered. Although the biopsy reveals a DCIS, there may be areas of carcinoma in the solid tumour that were missed and hence complete excision along with a sentinel node sampling is recommended.

21   C

Propylthiouracil is the treatment of choice in the management of hyperthyroidism in pregnant and lactating women. Carbimazole and iodine therapy may be considered after cessation of breastfeeding; however, one should not encourage the mother to stop breastfeeding. Atenolol is also contraindicated in breastfeeding women.

22   D

Cushing's disease is due to a pituitary adenoma, which secretes ACTH. The resulting clinical picture is no different from Cushing's syndrome. However, the plasma ACTH is raised in contrast to an adrenal adenoma or exogenous source where the plasma ACTH is lowered owing to the negative feedback of cortisol on the pituitary.

23   C

The commonest site of vascular aneurysms is the abdominal aorta. Following this, the commonest site of peripheral vascular aneurysms is the popliteal artery followed by the femoral artery. Although rare, the commonest site of abdominal vascular aneurysms is the splenic artery.

24   D

Arteries have been shown to have better outcomes than veins for their use in bypass procedures. Before superficial veins are harvested for use, a deep vein thrombosis must be excluded. An Allen's time of 15 seconds indicates that the radial artery may be the only main blood supply to the hand, in which case removing of it may render the hand ischaemic. Before veins are used, they may need to be stripped of any valves inside and reversed to act as a conduit, otherwise an immediate blockage of flow may occur.

25   E

Cushing's ulcer – stress ulceration from head injuries

Venous ulcer – lipodermatosclerosis and haemosiderin deposits

Curling's ulcer – stress ulcer from burns

Neuropathic ulcer – diabetes

Marjolin's ulcer – squamous cell carcinoma occurring in a chronic ulcer or scar tissue.

26   C

Nervous tissue is the most sensitive tissue in the human body to hypoxaemia and can undergo irreversible ischaemic changes within minutes of being deprived of oxygen.

27   D

The left kidney is the kidney of choice as it has the longer renal vein (the cava being to the right of the aorta). A BMI of 31 is not an absolute contraindication to donation; GFR of 110 mL/min is within the normal range for his age. It is possible for siblings not to have HLA antigens in common. The proof for consanguinity is to check the parents' HLA type or the HLA type of other siblings.

28   D

Bony fixation needs to be done first as this will act as the strut for the finger re-implantation. After this the venous return is established as this can often be the most difficult part of the operation and, if the veins are damaged beyond repair or avulsed, then there would be no point in establishing arterial continuity. The artery is then re-anastomosed on one side as this is often adequate and then the nerves and tendons may be repaired. The skin is finally closed last.

29   C

For intracapsular fracture fixation in the presence of good quality bone, the best method of fixation is with cannulated screws. The majority of patients are elderly with osteoporotic bone; therefore a hemiarthroplasty is performed. A dynamic hip screw is usually performed for extracapsular fractures.

30   D

The commonest cause for pain after a manipulation is because of swelling and a tight cast. It is important to keep the limb elevated to reduce the swelling and split the cast. Delay can lead to limb ischaemia and muscle damage resulting in ischaemic contractures. If a patient undergoes an open reduction and there are median nerve symptoms at presentation, then a carpal tunnel decompression can be done at the same time.

31   D

The musculocutaneous nerve pierces the coracobrachialis 5–8 cm distal to the coracoid process. This nerve gives branches to the coracobrachialis muscle, the biceps brachii and the brachialis muscles. The elbow joint is supplied by this nerve before it becomes the lateral cutaneous nerve of the forearm.

32   B

Usually the L4/5 disc is involved followed closely by the L5/S1. Most herniations are posterolateral and patients present with symptoms of backache and sciatica. Acute central disc herniations can cause a cauda equina compression syndrome. In a classical syndrome the patient has pain at the backs of thighs and legs; numbness in the buttocks, perineum and soles of feet; weakness/paralysis of legs and feet; and dysfunction of the bladder and bowel.

33   A

Gallbladder tumours occur in the fundus in 60% of patients, in the body in 30% of patients, and in the neck in 10% of patients. They are rarely found in the UK and are associated with gallstones and porcelain gallbladders.

34   E

Herceptin is the first humanised antibody (immunotherapy) approved for the treatment of HER2-positive metastatic breast cancer. Herceptin is designed to target and block the function of HER2 protein overexpression. Herceptin administration can result in the development of certain heart problems, including congestive heart failure. Severe allergic reactions, infusion reactions, and lung problems have been observed. Anaemia and leukopenia have also been reported when it is used in combination with chemotherapy.

35   E

Primary malignant bone tumours account for 1% of all deaths from malignant disease in the UK. The order of frequency of bone tumours from commonest to least is osteosarcoma, chondrosarcoma, and then Ewing's sarcoma. Pain and swelling are the commonest presenting features. Radiographic features of an osteosarcoma reveal a sclerotic intramedullary lesion of the metaphysis which expands and destroys the cortex. Unfortunately, by the time of presentation, over 90% of patients already have cortical destruction.

36   D

Double-lumen endotracheal tubes are essential for any cardiothoracic or oesophageal procedure to allow control of individual lungs during surgery and to avoid damaging lungs while the chest is opened.

37   B

Blind nasotracheal intubation is contraindicated in apnoea. Any nasotracheal intubation is contraindicated if a basal skull fracture is suspected from head or facial trauma. C-spine injury on its own is not a contraindication, especially in a breathing patient.

38   C

Vocal cord paralysis only occurs with direct trauma to the cords or damage to the recurrent laryngeal nerves. A surgical cricothyroidotomy does not involve direct trauma to the cord or nerves because the incision occurs at the cricothyroid membrane.

39   D

This scenario is demonstrating a Class III haemorrhage in which there is tachycardia >120/min, a reduced blood pressure and urine output, and an increased respiratory rate >30. Class III haemorrhage involves a blood loss of between 1.5–2 L.

40   E

Volume replacement in the trauma setting uses the 3 for 1 replacement rule with crystalloids. Ideally for Class III haemorrhage, blood replacement should be given as soon as possible. In the meanwhile, the volume of crystalloid should be replaced with 3 L for every litre of blood lost.

41   B

Laryngectomy is classed as a clean-contaminated procedure as it involves entering the airways and coming into contact with such pathogens. Examples of procedures are listed below:

- clean procedure – thyroidectomy
- clean-contaminated procedure – cholecystectomy
- contaminated procedure – right hemicolectomy
- dirty procedure – perforated colon/faecal peritonitis.

42   C

Iodine solutions have a very broad spectrum disinfecting activity, especially when compared with chlorhexidine. Unfortunately, iodine is easily deactivated when in contact with organic solutions such as bodily fluids. Chlorhexidine is less irritating to the skin and has a longer duration of action than does iodine.

43   A

An appendicectomy should be carried out if the patient agrees with the treatment and is competent to make that choice. In this case, she takes priority over her parent's wishes. For children under 16, they may consent to treatment if they are deemed competent to understand the procedure, risks and complications.

44   C

Monopolar diathermy uses a very high-frequency alternating current at high voltages to cut and coagulate tissue using the patient as a circuit where the active end acts as a current density channel. Cutting is accomplished by a continuous wave output of current whereas coagulation uses a pulsed output to help cool tissues while heating them and results in a coagulum rather than complete destruction.

45   D

Capacitance coupling occurs with the use of insulated instruments and combining plastic and metal ports with instruments when laparoscopic surgery is being performed. The combined energy is insulated as the metal–plastic–metal layering acts as a capacitor. Such coupling can be avoided by a high index of suspicion and vigilance over the use of port and instrument combinations. Use of all similar ports avoids capacitance and coupling.

46   D

Standard HIV precautions exist to minimise any chance of inoculation from blood contact. Double gloving, disposable gowns, and kidney dish passing of sharp instruments are just some of the few precautions listed. There are no suggestions for specific theatre ventilation in HIV as this is not transmitted via airborne routes.

47   C

The anion gap would be increased in conditions where unmeasured anions exist in the blood in metabolic acidosis. Examples include lactic acidosis, ketones from diabetic ketoacidosis, and drugs that may be taken in overdose. Diarrhoea and loss of bicarbonate do not result in an increased anion gap.

48   E

Thrombophlebitis does not usually occur in such large bore veins. It is recognised in peripheral veins with the use of hyperosmolar solutions; however, this is the exact reason why a central vein is used instead.

49   B

The priority in the management of burns is to remove the source of burns and then systematically resuscitate the victim starting with airway, breathing and circulation. All burns are painful. Although full thickness burns may have a central area of painless tissue because of burnt nerves, there is a transition area around the edges from surrounding normal skin and areas of lesser degree burns, which will be very sensitive. Fluid replacement in burns uses a formula that does not incorporate the degree of burns as a factor; however, percentage area burned and body weight are key factors.

50   D

Refeeding syndrome occurs when previously malnourished patients are fed with high loads of carbohydrate, resulting in a rapid fall in phosphate, magnesium, potassium, and calcium levels, along with an increasing ECF volume and subsequent hyponatraemia. Hypoglycaemia is not a key feature of the refeeding syndrome although may be seen if the insulin response is oversensitive. Initial hyperglycaemia is the norm as a high-carbohydrate diet is fed.

51   E

It may be difficult to quantify exactly how much aspirin has been overdosed in this clinical scenario; however, a fair number is suspected as the patient is complaining of new onset tinnitus. It is not unusual for many patients to take an overdose and start vomiting a considerable amount. The initial aspirin absorption would result in an anion-gap metabolic acidosis. The resultant vomiting would cause a metabolic alkalosis, hence leading to the combined picture as seen here, despite the blood gas results being fairly normal values. Interpretation of blood gas results requires putting the entire clinical picture together. In aspirin overdose, a respiratory alkalosis may also been seen if the patient starts to hyperventilate, which is not uncommon.

52   D

Most patients post laparotomy for upper GI surgery will have some ventilatory difficulties from the postoperative incision pain. This could result in a respiratory acidosis from hypoventilation as indicated by the high pCO_2 value. A normal pH and high bicarbonate in this instance suggests a compensatory response.

53   A

This diabetic patient has been starving for their procedure in the day case unit. The blood gas results show a clear metabolic acidosis from the low pH, low HCO_3, and normal pCO_2. One must assume that this is due to diabetic ketoacidosis, which would result in an anion-gap metabolic acidosis owing to the ketones present acting as unmeasured anions.

54   B

Peutz–Jehger's disease is an autosomal dominant disorder characterised by the presence of hamartomatous polyps within the GI tract as well as circumoral pigmentation. Examples of metaplasia include Barratt's oesophagus and squamous change of the cervix, bronchus, or bladder. Examples of dysplasia include cervical intra-epithelial neoplasia (CIN) and vulvar intra-epithelial neoplasia (VIN). Paget's disease and FAP are examples of neoplastic disorders.

55   E

Fistulae-in-ano may form from any infection or systemic irritation occurring around the anus. Examples include neoplasia, inflammatory bowel disease, foreign bodies, and radiation damage. Inadequate vascularisation does not predispose to the development of a fistula, although it may prevent its healing.

56   D

FAP accounts for <1% of colorectal cancers and is characterised by the development of hundreds to thousands of polyps within the colon and rectum. It is inherited as an autosomal dominant condition, although some cases may arise from a de-novo mutation of the long arm of the chromosome 5 where the gene is located. Cancers develop in the 4th and 5th decades typically and this condition is associated with a 100% lifetime risk of developing cancer. Affected individuals are treated with a prophylactic total or subtotal colectomy.

57   E

Complement functions are as follows:

- **Opsonisation** – C3b
- **Chemotaxis** – C5a and C5, C6, C7
- **Anaphylatoxin** – C3a<C4a<C5a
- **Cytolysis** – C5b6789 complex

58   E

Multiple endocrine neoplasia (MEN) type 1 is an uncommon inherited disorder affecting the parathyroid, pituitary and pancreas. Occasionally adrenal cortical disorders may also occur as part of the syndrome. Phaeochromocytomas are associated with MEN type 2 variety.

59   B

White pulp consists of central arteries ensheathed by lymphoid nodules and lymphocytes. White pulp contains T lymphocytes located immediately in the vicinity of the central artery. Most of the antibody synthesis in the spleen occurs in the white pulp. Red pulp forms most of the splenic volume and contains sinusoids, which trap defective red cells.

60   A

The quiescent or G_0 phase is the dormant phase of the cell cycle where no cell division takes place, although cells are still capable of undergoing mitosis. It is this phase of the cell cycle that is most resistant to chemotherapeutic agents. Most chemotherapeutic agents produce their lethal effect on cells that are actively replicating. Higher doses of chemotherapeutic agents are required to target cells in this phase of the cycle.

61   E

Dobutamine acts on both $\alpha 1$ and $\beta 1$ adrenergic receptors as an agonist, although the racemic mixture contains some $\alpha 1$-antagonist activity as well. Dobutamine is used clinically for its $\beta 1$ activity in increasing cardiac contractility in congestive cardiac failure preferably owing to non-ischaemic causes.

62   C

Gastrin is secreted from the G cells in response to ACh stimulation to act on the parietal cells and cause acid release. Histamine is released from the enterochromaffin cells in response to ACh to act directly on the parietal cells like gastrin. The three phases of gastric secretion include cephalic 30%, gastric 65% and intestinal 5% phases.

63   E

Colonic flora comprises a huge population of both aerobic and anaerobic bacteria. They are involved in:

- fermentation of indigestible carbohydrates and production of fatty acids that the colonic mucosa may use as an energy source
- degradation of bilirubin to stercobilin, urobilin, and urobilinogen
- synthesis of vitamins B_1, B_2, B_{12}, and vitamin K.

64   D

Osmoreceptors stimulate ADH release from the posterior pituitary in response to increases in extracellular fluid osmolality. ADH secretion is also stimulated by a decrease in blood pressure or decreased circulating volume. ADH serves to increase the water permeability in the distal tubule and collecting ducts in addition to increasing the arterial blood pressure by causing peripheral vasoconstriction.

65   B

Average values of secreted fluids include:

Mouth	1.5 L saliva secreted
Stomach	2–3 L secreted
Gallbladder	500 mL secreted
Pancreas	1.5 L secreted
Small bowel	1.5 L secreted
Large bowel	100 mL excreted

66   A

α1-antitrypsin deficiency causes emphysema, which results an increased compliance of the lung tissue. All of the other listed conditions decrease lung compliance.

67   A

Hypoxia and hypercapnia both cause constriction of the smaller alveolar vessel and thus divert blood to areas that are better oxygenated. This is in contrast to peripheral vessels where the opposite response is seen and hypoxia causes vasodilatation. The ideal area for ventilation and perfusion matching (V/Q = 1) within the lung occurs about two-thirds of the way up from the base of the lung.

68   D

Fetal haemoglobin (HbF), is made up of 2-α globin and 2-δ globulins. This difference in globin structure, makes HbF unable to react with 2,3-DPG and thus has a higher affinity for oxygen for a given PO_2. This ensures that oxygen is transferred from the maternal blood to the fetal blood, regardless of the PO_2 in the maternal blood. In comparison with the dissociation curve of adult haemoglobin, that of HbF is shifted to the left. It is also found in higher proportions in the blood of those individuals affected with sickle-cell anaemia or thalassaemia such as Arabian or African populations.

69   B

Atrial natriuretic peptide (ANP) is a 28-amino acid peptide that is synthesised, stored, and released by atrial cells in response to atrial distension, angiotensin II and sympathetic stimulation (β-adrenoceptor mediated). Elevated levels of ANP are found during hypervolaemic states and congestive heart failure. ANP serves to increase the GFR and inhibit the tubular resorption of Na^+. The end result leads to an increase in sodium and water excretion.

70   C

This patient is presented with symptomatic and prolapsing piles. Treatment by injection and banding or conservative management is unlikely to deal ideally with the entire problem. The procedure for prolapse and haemorrhoidopexy (PPH) is the best option from the listed choices in this case. A Delorme procedure is the operation that employs the perineal approach to reduce a full thickness bowel prolapse and is not indicated.

71   D

Gardner's syndrome and FAP share the same APC gene that mutates on the long arm of chromosome 5. Risk factors for colon cancer include genetic causes, diet, irradiation, surgical procedures and inflammatory bowel disease. Cancers occurring post ureterosigmoidostomy classically occurs at or near the ureterocolic anastomosis. Interestingly, around two-thirds of cancers are proximal to the splenic flexure in HNPCC.

72   A

5-FU is commonly used in the adjuvant chemotherapy in managing colorectal cancers. Colorectal cancers should be treated with excision where possible, although in some cases a limited case of pre-operative chemo-radiotherapy may be required. The management of ascending colon tumour in the acute obstructed setting would include a right hemicolectomy plus a defunctioning loop ileostomy and not a colostomy. Surveillance colonoscopy should be performed for the first 5–10 years every 2 years and not annually, although local guidelines may differ slightly. There is no difference shown from numerous studies that there is any difference between hand-sewn and stapled bowel anastomoses.

73   E

Diverticular disease is more prevalent in the developed world and theories suggest this may be due to a lack of dietary factors. Prevention and not resolution of diverticular disease may occur with the use of high fibre diets, which puts less strain on the colon theoretically. Once diverticular disease is established, only surgery may completely eradicate it; however, attacks of diverticulitis are usually managed conservatively unless these symptoms are troubling enough with frequent attacks or complications from the initial disease have occurred (fistula or abscess formation).

74   A

The commonest cause of small bowel obstruction is from adhesions within the peritoneal cavity. This usually results from previous abdominal surgery. The other causes listed are less common then adhesions and include an inguinal hernia, which may present as a lump in the groin above and medial to the pubic tubercle or femoral hernia, which lies below and lateral to the pubic tubercle. Circumoral pigmentation is suggestive of Peutz–Jegher's syndrome which may cause an intussusception from hamartomatous polyps in the small bowel. A nodule at the umbilicus in combination with cachexia is suggestive of a Sister Joseph's nodule, which may indicate an internal malignancy.

75   E

Zollinger–Ellison syndrome is caused by a gastrinoma, which results in excessive acid secretion owing to high levels of gastrin. A course of PPI will not cure the ulcer as cessation of therapy will result in recurrence. The definitive treatment is by surgical excision of the gastrinoma. All of the other causes listed may be cured by a course of PPI.

76   C

Renal artery stenosis is usually caused by a fibromuscular hyperplasia of the renal arteries rather than atherosclerosis in younger patients. Treatment options include surgery or dilatation and stenting under angiographic control.

77   C

This case presentation is highly suggestive of a testicular torsion. With the limited time in which to prevent testicular infarction, the management in this case without a doubt is urgent exploration of the testes in the operating theatre. Any investigation would delay the diagnosis and possibly lead to an unviable testis at surgery. Ideally these cases should be operated on as soon as possible but most definitely within 6 hours of onset. After this time irreversible changes may occur, and an orchidectomy should also be considered as a likely possibility.

78   D

Urethral strictures can be managed with urethral catheterisation. However, this is not a form definitive treatment.

79   D

Boundaries of the epiploic foramen of Winslow include:

- **Anteriorly:** free edge of the lesser omentum containing the porta hepatis
- **Posteriorly:** IVC
- **Superiorly:** caudate process of liver
- **Inferiorly:** first part of duodenum.

80   D

The Pfannensteil incision is a low-lying transverse incision commonly used in open gynaecological and obstetric procedures. Although the initial skin incision is transverse, the rectus muscle is opened vertically in the line of the linea alba. The skin and two layers of subcutaneous tissue (Camper's and Scarpa's fascia) are incised as well as the linea alba and its overlying anterior rectus sheath to which it is fused. The peritoneum is the next encountered layer as the posterior rectus sheath is deficient below the level of the arcuate line, located roughly halfway between the pubis and umbilicus.

81   C

An standard right hemicolectomy may endanger the right ureter, right gonadal artery and vein, and the second part of the duodenum. When this is made into an extended right hemicolectomy, the spleen may also be damaged as part of the mobilisation. The fourth part of the duodenum is relatively safe in this procedure as it lies near the ligament of Treitz.

82   D

Differences between jejunum and ileum are as follows:

	Jejunum	Ileum
Position	Upper left abdomen	Lower right abdomen
Extent	2/5	3/5
External feel and appearance	Thick, wide, vascular	Thin, narrow, pale
Peyer's patches	Few	Many
Vascular arcades	Few	Many
Vasa recti	Long	Short
Mesenteric fat	Less	More

83   B

Suprascapular nerve injury is a rare clinical syndrome, but may arise in volleyball players and those undergoing radical neck dissection for malignancy. The supraspinatus and infraspinatus muscles are affected and initiation of abduction is weakened.

84   D

Adductor pollicis muscle is supplied by the ulnar nerve as well as most intrinsic muscles of the hand. Within the hand, the median nerve supplies the LOAF muscles, which include: lateral two lumbricals, opponens pollicis, abductor pollicis brevis, and flexor pollicis brevis.

85   C

The suprascapular artery is a branch of the thyrocervical trunk of the subclavian artery. All of the others listed are direct branches of the axillary artery in addition to the anterior and posterior circumflex humeral arteries from the third part.

86   E

The trachea is lined by ciliated columnar epithelium and commences at the level of the cricoid cartilage (C6) and ends at the carina (T4/5), which is also the level of the 2nd costal cartilage extending into the 2nd rib.

87   C

The left recurrent laryngeal nerve may be damaged in thoracic surgery as it ascends from the vagus nerve and hooks around the ligamentum arteriosum to carry on cranially and supply the extrinsic muscles of the larynx. Damage to this nerve would result in a unilateral vocal cord palsy and hence hoarseness of voice.

88   B

Pectineus is a medial rotator of the hip joint. It arises from the pectineal line of the pubis and a small area on the superior pubic ramus just below it and attaches to a vertical line below the lesser trochanter of the femur. The nerve supply is from the anterior division of the femoral nerve, although it may occasionally receive a twig from the obturator nerve as well.

89   C

Meniscal injuries classically arise when a large force is applied to the knee in a semi-flexed position. The medial cartilage is more commonly damaged than the lateral one owing to anatomical reasons of size, location and mobility. Cruciate injuries result from hyperextension of the knee and result in instability rather than locking as found in meniscal tears.

90   D

The tendon of obturator internus and its corresponding nerve pass through the lesser sciatic foramen as well as the pudendal nerve and internal pudendal vessels. The other structures listed all pass through the greater sciatic foramen only.

PRACTICE PAPER 3: QUESTIONS

PRACTICE PAPER 3: QUESTIONS

1 A 55-year-old man presents to you with back pain and paraesthesia along the medial border of the leg and foot. A disc prolapse is suspected with compression of which of the following spinal nerve roots?

○ A L3

○ B L4

○ C L5

○ D S1

○ E S2

2 All of the following muscles are involved in abduction of the hip joint EXCEPT

○ A gluteus medius

○ B gluteus minimus

○ C sartorius

○ D quadratus femoris

○ E tensor fasciae latae

3   An obese 45-year-old waitress is referred to you by her GP with a diagnosis of meralgia paraesthetica. You would expect her symptoms to affect which of the following areas?

○   A   gluteal region

○   B   posterior thigh

○   C   anterolateral thigh

○   D   medial thigh

○   E   groin area

4   Which of the following veins accompanies the marginal branch of the right coronary artery?

○   A   great cardiac vein

○   B   middle cardiac vein

○   C   small cardiac vein

○   D   anterior cardiac vein

○   E   oblique cardiac vein

5   A 52-year-old businessman is admitted to A&E with acute onset chest pain, which radiates to the right arm and is associated with nausea and sweating. An ECG taken shows ischaemic changes within the heart and you suspect that he has angina. Transmission of activity within which of the following afferent nerves would explain the pain radiating down the arm from the chest?

⭕ A   phrenic nerve

⭕ B   vagus nerve

⭕ C   somatic nerves to the arm

⭕ D   intercostal nerves

⭕ E   splanchnic nerves

6   All of the following structures would drain through the thoracic duct EXCEPT

⭕ A   left arm and thorax

⭕ B   left face and neck

⭕ C   left side of abdomen

⭕ D   right face and neck

⭕ E   right side of abdomen

7   Innervation to the muscles of the back originate from

⭕ A   dorsal primary rami

⭕ B   ventral primary rami

⭕ C   grey rami communicantes

⭕ D   white rami communicantes

⭕ E   lateral perforating branches of the ventral primary rami

8 **Which of the following nerves provides the afferent limb of the sneezing reflex?**

  ○ A ophthalmic division of the trigeminal nerve

  ○ B maxillary division of the trigeminal nerve

  ○ C mandibular division of the trigeminal nerve

  ○ D glossopharyngeal nerve

  ○ E vagus nerve

9 **A 44-year-old-man presents to you with signs of a facial infection around the area of the pterygopalatine fossa following maxillary surgery. You initially suspect that the infection has tracked from the pterygoid venous plexus. All of the following structures are at risk of subsequent infection tracking down EXCEPT**

  ○ A orbit

  ○ B oral cavity

  ○ C nasal cavity

  ○ D maxillary sinus

  ○ E middle cranial fossa

10 **All of the following nerves pass along the lateral wall of the cavernous sinus EXCEPT**

  ○ A oculomotor nerve

  ○ B trochlear nerve

  ○ C ophthalmic division of the trigeminal nerve

  ○ D maxillary division of the trigeminal nerve

  ○ E abducent nerve

11 All of the following statements regarding the chemical control of respiration are correct EXCEPT

○ A   the carotid bodies are sensitive to hypoxaemia

○ B   the carotid bodies are sensitive to hypercapnia

○ C   the central medullary chemoreceptors are sensitive to hypoxaemia

○ D   the central medullary chemoreceptors are sensitive to hypercapnia

○ E   the central medullary chemoreceptors are sensitive to changes in H^+

12 A 28-year-old woman gives birth to a healthy baby girl in the delivery suite. During her 2nd stage of labour an episiotomy was necessary to allow delivery of her baby under local anaesthesia. Immediately after this procedure, the woman now complains that she is unable to maintain continence of faeces as she has no voluntary control of her anal sphincters. Which nerve in this clinical scenario has been anaesthetised?

○ A   pudendal nerve

○ B   inferior gluteal nerve

○ C   superior gluteal nerve

○ D   ventral rami of S3 and S4

○ E   inferior hypogastric nerve

13   **The lateral umbilical folds in the abdominal wall are formed by**

○   A   urachus

○   B   obliterated umbilical arteries

○   C   superior epigastric arteries

○   D   inferior epigastric arteries

○   E   falciform ligament

14   **A bleeding ulcer on the posterior aspect of the first part of the duodenum would classically erode through which of the following vessels?**

○   A   right gastric artery

○   B   superior pancreaticoduodenal artery

○   C   right gastroepiploic artery

○   D   gastroduodenal artery

○   E   hepatic artery

15   **The developmental origin of the uterus and uterine tubes are the**

○   A   pronephric ducts

○   B   mesonephric ducts

○   C   metanephric ducts

○   D   paramesonephric ducts

○   E   Wolffian ducts

16   Cerebrospinal fluid is connected to the subarachnoid space from the ventricles via the

○   A   cisterna magna

○   B   arachnoid villi

○   C   choroid plexus

○   D   foramen of Monro

○   E   foramina of Magendie and Luschka

17   All of the following statements regarding malignant hyperpyrexia are true EXCEPT

○   A   relatives of affected individuals should always be tested

○   B   inheritance in an autosomal recessive pattern

○   C   incidence is 1 in 200,000

○   D   treatment involves the use of dantrolene sodium and fluids

○   E   conclusive diagnosis requires a muscle biopsy in addition to the clinical picture

18   Which of the following statements regarding immunosuppressive drugs used in renal transplantation is correct?

○   A   azathioprine is more effective than mycophenolate in preventing acute rejection

○   B   tacrolimus works by directly inhibiting nucleic acid synthesis

○   C   mycophenolate works by inhibiting enzymes in the pathway for purine synthesis

○   D   sirolimus has greater nephrotoxicity than cyclosporine

○   E   basiliximab is not commonly used as an induction agent in renal transplants

19 The main host defences against bacterial exotoxins in a person with an intact immunological system are

○ A T-helper cells

○ B T-cytotoxic cells

○ C activated macrophages that secrete proteases

○ D IgM and IgG antibodies

○ E host-cell receptor modulation in response to toxins

20 All of the following statements regarding interferons are correct EXCEPT they

○ A are induced by dsRNA

○ B are typically specific to their host species cell of origin

○ C appear typically before antibodies in viral infections

○ D inhibit the growth of both DNA and RNA viruses

○ E enhance the metabolism of infected cells

21 Which of the following statements regarding the hepatitis B virus (HBV) is correct?

○ A HBV belongs to the Picornaviridae group of viruses

○ B hepatitis B may not be transmitted via breast milk

○ C 25% of patients infected with hepatitis B become chronic carriers

○ D risk of transmission from needlestick injuries is greater for HBV than HIV

○ E HBV vaccines are live-attenuated vaccines

22 A 23-year-old male is brought into A&E after having sustained three stab wounds to the abdomen with evisceration of small bowel. A laparotomy is performed where gross faecal contamination is found from large bowel lacerations. The bowel injuries are resected and a defunctioning ileostomy is performed. On the 4th postoperative day, the patient becomes develops a temperature of 39°C with peritonitis as well as buttock myonecrosis with foul smelling discharge. In this clinical scenario, which of the following organisms is most likely to cause this infection?

○ A *Helicobacter pylori*

○ B *Bacteroides fragilis*

○ C *Vibrio parahaemolyticus*

○ D *Salmonella typhi*

○ E *Shigella dysenteriae*

23 Indications for splenectomy include all of the following EXCEPT

○ A thrombotic thrombocytopenic purpura

○ B Felty's syndrome

○ C thrombocytopenia associated with drug abuse

○ D sickle cell disease without hypersplenism

○ E splenomegaly related to haemodialysis

24   The commonest infection to affect the asplenic patient following splenectomy is

○   A   *Streptococcus pneumoniae*

○   B   *Neisseria meningitides*

○   C   *Escherichia coli*

○   D   *Haemophilus influenzae*

○   E   *Staphylococcus aureus*

25   Clinical presentation of neurogenic shock include which of the following combination of signs?

○   A   hypotension, bradycardia, warm skin

○   B   hypotension, tachycardia, warm skin

○   C   hypotension, bradycardia, cool skin

○   D   hypotension, tachycardia, cool skin

○   E   hypertension, bradycardia, cool skin

26   Smoking causes all of the following physiological effects EXCEPT

○   A   a shift of the oxygen dissociation curve to the left

○   B   impaired wound healing and increased risk of wound breakdown

○   C   impaired mucociliary function

○   D   no change in cardiovascular function when stopped 1 day before surgery

○   E   an increase in pulse rate and mean arterial pressure

27   **All of the following statements regarding Swan–Ganz pulmonary artery catheters are true EXCEPT**

⃝   A   the insertion procedure may be complicated by arrhythmias

⃝   B   pulmonary arterial pressures readings of 6–12 mmHg are normal

⃝   C   left atrial pressure may be measured reasonably accurately

⃝   D   it can be used as part of the thermodilution mechanism to measure cardiac output accurately

⃝   E   it should always be inserted under strict septic technique

28   **Which of the following statements regarding suxamethonium is true?**

⃝   A   it is a non-depolarising muscle relaxant

⃝   B   it is not very useful in crash inductions

⃝   C   it is structurally similar to the acetylcholine molecule

⃝   D   prolonged action can be due to the presence of too much plasma cholinesterase

⃝   E   it has a half-life of 10 minutes, making it short acting

29 A 42-year old alcoholic man is referred to you with ascites and liver cirrhosis. The mechanism of formation of ascites in this patient with cirrhosis is a combination of which of the following conditions?

○ A hypoalbuminaemia and portal hypertension present
○ B decreased hepatic lymph flow
○ C decreased hepatic lymph flow with decreased aldosterone secretion
○ D leaky capillaries in the portal circulation
○ E sub-acute inflammatory changes causing hepatic oedema and extravasation of fluid

30 A 35-year old businessman presents to you for an endoscopy following symptoms of epigastric pain which is worse at nights and on eating food. You suspect a gastric ulcer and proceed to perform endoscopy with a biopsy for *Helicobacter pylori*. On endoscopic biopsy, which of the following is the commonest location for finding *Helicobacter pylori* within the stomach?

○ A fundus
○ B lesser curve
○ C body
○ D pyloric antrum
○ E cardia

31   Sick euthyroid syndrome consists of all of the following signs EXCEPT

○   A   decreased number of binding proteins

○   B   decreased affinity of binding proteins

○   C   decreased thyroid-stimulating hormone (TSH)

○   D   decreased peripheral conversion of T_3 to T_4

○   E   normal thyroid functioning

32   All of the following principles are used in the management of chronic renal failure EXCEPT

○   A   high dose loop diuretics in the management of hypertension

○   B   fluid restriction to prevent the development of oedema

○   C   sodium restriction to help limit fluid overload

○   D   high protein diet to prevent muscle atrophy in catabolism

○   E   calcium chloride to help bind gut phosphate in hyperphosphataemia

33   All of the following signs maybe produced by a Pancoast's tumour at the apex of the right lung EXCEPT

○   A   oedema and venous engorgement of the right upper limb

○   B   hoarseness of voice

○   C   ipsilateral paradoxical diaphragmatic movement

○   D   hyperhidrosis of the right side of the face

○   E   enophthalmos and miosis in the right eye

34 Which of the following structures may be injured in supracondylar fracture of the femur?

- ○ A sciatic nerve
- ○ B popliteal artery
- ○ C long saphenous vein
- ○ D short saphenous vein
- ○ E deep femoral artery

35 All of the following muscles are supplied by the posterior interosseous branch of the radial nerve EXCEPT

- ○ A extensor carpi radialis longus
- ○ B extensor digitorum
- ○ C extensor digiti minimi
- ○ D abductor pollicis longus
- ○ E extensor pollicis brevis

36 Which of the following statements regarding the triquetral bone is correct?

- ○ A the degree of contact with the radioulnar articular disc is maximal in full adduction of the wrist joint
- ○ B it lies just laterally to the lunate bone
- ○ C it forms part of the radiocarpal joint in the wrist
- ○ D the hamate lies just anterolaterally to the triquetral
- ○ E during forced hyperextension of the wrist joint, anterior dislocation of the triquetral can cause carpal tunnel syndrome

37   A 23-year-old man undergoes open reduction and internal fixation of the right tibia after having sustained injuries from a road traffic accident. Shortly after his return to the ward, he begins to complain of paraesthesia in his toes as well as pain in his right leg, which is not relieved by analgesia. He has good distal pulses and sensation to his right foot. The first step in the management of this patient would be to

○   A   measure his compartment pressures in the right leg

○   B   prescribe stronger analgesia as this is a common postoperative complaint

○   C   call your seniors as he may have a trapped nerve from the surgery

○   D   book theatres immediately for urgent fasciotomies as you are highly suspicious of compartment syndrome

○   E   split the cast to relieve any pressure from postoperative swelling and reassess the situation in 10 minutes

38   Drainage of the right testicular vein normally occurs into the

○   A   portal vein

○   B   inferior vena cava

○   C   right renal vein

○   D   right internal iliac vein

○   E   right suprarenal vein

39   The CHARGE syndrome is NOT associated which of the following conditions?

○ A   choanal atresia

○ B   genital abnormalities

○ C   facial nerve palsy

○ D   retarded lung maturation

○ E   coloboma

40   Which of these conditions does NOT predispose towards acute sinusitis?

○ A   immunocompromisation

○ B   dental infection

○ C   nasal polyposis

○ D   Kartagener's syndrome

○ E   Waardenberg's syndrome

41   Which of the following is NOT a complication of tracheostomy?

○ A   tracheal necrosis

○ B   recurrent laryngeal nerve injury

○ C   pneumothorax

○ D   hypothyroidism

○ E   tracheocutaneous fistula

42   **The most common site affected in oral cavity carcinoma is**

- ○   A   hard palate
- ○   B   lateral border of the tongue
- ○   C   tonsils
- ○   D   buccal mucosa
- ○   E   soft palate

43   **A 50-year-old woman is found to be febrile one day after her total gastrectomy for malignancy. The most likely cause of this is**

- ○   A   urinary tract infection
- ○   B   pulmonary embolus
- ○   C   wound infection
- ○   D   anastomotic leak
- ○   E   atelectasis

44   **Concerning laparoscopic surgery which of the following is NOT true?**

- ○   A   shoulder tip pain is a common postoperative complaint
- ○   B   bowel perforation should have consent
- ○   C   Verres needles should be inserted under direct vision
- ○   D   conduction coupling is a recognised risk
- ○   E   pneumoperitoneum may lead to pneumomediastinum

45 **The following vessels all supply blood to the oesophagus EXCEPT**

- A   inferior thyroid artery
- B   inferior phrenic artery
- C   left gastric artery branches
- D   superior phrenic artery
- E   aortic and bronchial branches

46 **High anal fistulae**

- A   are more common than low anal fistulae
- B   open into the rectum above the puborectalis muscle
- C   can be managed with a loose seton
- D   are typically associated with ulcerative colitis
- E   may be laid open without hazard

47 **Which of the following is true of ulcerative colitis?**

- A   it is commonly associated with anal fistulae
- B   it is commonly associated with oral ulceration
- C   it is worsened by smoking
- D   it is associated with abdominal masses
- E   it is associated with joint pain

48   **The following statements about hernias are all true EXCEPT**

○   A   direct hernias are due to a deficiency at Hesselbach's triangle

○   B   a Littre's hernia contains a Meckel's diverticulum

○   C   a femoral hernia usually presents as a lump above and lateral to the pubic tubercle

○   D   Richter's hernia involves entrapment of the antimesenteric edge of the bowel

○   E   Spigelian hernias protrude from the lateral edge of the rectus abdominis muscle

49   **High output stomas are associated with the following EXCEPT**

○   A   distal position

○   B   electrolyte disturbances

○   C   diarrhoea

○   D   octreotide to reduce output

○   E   loperamide to reduce output

50   **The following are known to cause a metabolic acidosis EXCEPT**

○   A   myocardial infarction

○   B   ischaemic bowel

○   C   diabetic ketoacidosis

○   D   sepsis

○   E   persistent vomiting

51   **The following brachial plexus injuries would all give rise to the accompanying deficits EXCEPT**

○   A   radial nerve lesion – wrist drop

○   B   ulnar nerve lesion – claw deformity

○   C   axillary nerve injury – insensate shoulder patch

○   D   median nerve palsy – weakened thumb movements + loss of sensation to lateral palm

○   E   thoracodorsal nerve injury – winged scapula

52   **Colonic diverticular disease**

○   A   may present with a colovesical fistula

○   B   does not present with colonic obstruction

○   C   is an inherited condition

○   D   is a premalignant condition

○   E   is not a feature of ageing

53   **The inguinal canal**

○   A   is approximately 2.5 cm long

○   B   has the fascia transversalis covering its whole posterior wall

○   C   has an internal ring lying 5 cm above the middle of the inguinal ligament

○   D   has the lacunar ligament in the medial part of its floor

○   E   has the inferior epigastric artery lying medial to its deep ring

54 **Which of the following stoma complications makes closure technically easier?**

○   A   parastomal hernia

○   B   prolapse

○   C   stenosis

○   D   retraction

○   E   ischaemia

55 **A 47-year-old male patient received a cadaver kidney transplant with immediate function 2 weeks ago. Within 3 days his serum creatinine had normalised to 110 μmol/L. He was discharged on the 5th postoperative day and has been followed up at the transplant follow-up clinic, attending thrice weekly. On attendance today his serum creatinine is 167 μmol/L and he is well in himself with no symptoms. You note on checking the blood results that the creatinine was 115 μmol/L two days ago. His tacrolimus (immunosuppression drug) level is normal. Ultrasound scan shows a normal transplant kidney. What is the most likely cause of his raised serum creatinine?**

○   A   acute rejection episode and a transplant biopsy is urgently required to confirm the diagnosis

○   B   acute tubular necrosis

○   C   volume depletion owing to diarrhoea and vomiting

○   D   ureteric obstruction

○   E   transplant renal artery stenosis

56   Bowel obstruction may be caused by all of the following EXCEPT

- ◯ A   volvulus
- ◯ B   hiatus herniae
- ◯ C   adhesions from previous surgery
- ◯ D   intussception
- ◯ E   polyp

57   All of the following statements regarding the management of trauma in pregnant women are true EXCEPT

- ◯ A   a qualified surgeon and obstetrician should always be consulted early in the evaluation of the pregnant patient
- ◯ B   small bowel injury in commoner in upper abdominal penetrating wounds than lower penetrating injuries in late pregnancy
- ◯ C   pregnant women show earlier signs of hypovolaemia during haemorrhage
- ◯ D   unless contraindicated, pregnant women should be placed in the left lateral position during assessment and management as early as possible
- ◯ E   all Rh-ve pregnant patients should be considered for Rh immunoglobulin therapy in penetrating abdominal injuries

58 All of the following may be considered risk factors for compartment syndrome in trauma EXCEPT

○ A severe crush injury to muscles

○ B ischaemic reperfusion to limb muscles

○ C flexion–distraction spinal injuries

○ D presence of limb burns

○ E immobilisation of injuries in tight casts and dressings

59 Complications of intraosseous needle puncture in children include all of the following EXCEPT

○ A physeal plate injury

○ B skin pressure necrosis

○ C subperiosteal infiltration

○ D musculocutaneous fistula

○ E osteomyelitis

60 Which of the following volumes of blood loss would accurately fall into a Class II haemorrhage?

○ A 500 mL

○ B 700 mL

○ C 1000 mL

○ D 1500 mL

○ E 2000 mL

61   **Causes of spontaneous secondary pneumothorax include all of the following EXCEPT**

○   A   Marfan's syndrome

○   B   lung cancer

○   C   asthma

○   D   COPD

○   E   lung abscesses

62   **All of the following statements regarding dead space ventilation are correct EXCEPT**

○   A   dead space refers to air that has to be ventilated, but does not take part in gas exchange

○   B   anatomical dead space refers to air that does not reach the alveoli to take place in ventilation

○   C   anatomical dead space can be measured using Fowler's method

○   D   physiological dead space maybe increased in positive pressure ventilation

○   E   anatomical dead space is reduced in the standing-up position

63   **Which of the following conditions would result in a positive base excess on a blood gas report?**

○   A   Cushing's syndrome

○   B   starvation

○   C   septicaemia

○   D   pulmonary embolus

○   E   myasthenia gravis

64   Fever may be caused by all of the following EXCEPT

○   A   heatstroke

○   B   hyperthyroidism

○   C   posterior hypothalamic lesions

○   D   dehydration

○   E   exercise

65   All of the following features are found in ARDS EXCEPT

○   A   pulmonary oedema of non-cardiogenic origin

○   B   hypoxaemia that is refractory to oxygen therapy

○   C   reduced lung compliance

○   D PaO_2/FiO_2 ratio <26.6 kPa (200 mmHg)

○   E   pulmonary capillary wedge pressure >16 mmHg

66   Which of the following features are found with a large pulmonary embolus?

○   A   decreased pulmonary vascular resistance

○   B   pulmonary hypertension

○   C   increased left ventricular output

○   D   decreased right ventricular afterload

○   E   increased lung compliance

67 A 43-year-old female patient has had a successful kidney transplant and is being discharged on the 5th postoperative day. One of the instructions she was given was not to eat grapefruit or drink grapefruit juice. This is because

○ A grapefruit juice has large amounts of potassium

○ B grapefruit juice is sour and may interfere with the patient's digestion

○ C grapefruit juice may interfere with the metabolism of tacrolimus, one of the immunosuppressive agents being used

○ D grapefruit juice may interact with the action of the statin that has been prescribed for her hypercholesterolaemia

○ E grapefruit juice may cause diarrhoea and interfere with the patient's fluid balance

68 A 57-year-old man was admitted to neurointensive care after a subarachnoid haemorrhage. He is not brainstem dead, but the neurosurgeon is of the opinion that further treatment is futile. His longstanding partner of 15 years, a 55-year-old man, is in agreement that treatment should be withdrawn. Which of the following statements is true?

○ A the patient cannot be a kidney donor because he is gay

○ B the patient cannot be a kidney donor because he is not brainstem dead

○ C the patient cannot be a donor because he is too old

○ D the patient is a potential non-heart beating donor of his liver and kidneys

○ E organ retrieval from such a patient is illegal

69   **Which of the following phases are correctly matched with their physiological action within the cardiac ventricular muscle action potential graph?**

○   A   Phase 0 – resting membrane potential

○   B   Phase 1 – rapid depolarisation

○   C   Phase 2 – slow depolarisation plateau

○   D   Phase 3 – rapid repolarisation

○   E   Phase 4 – slow repolarisation

70   **During observation of the venous pulse, you note that the *x*-descent is**

○   A   prominent in atrial systole

○   B   synchronous with the carotid pulse wave

○   C   reflects a rise in atrial pressure before the tricuspid valve opens

○   D   due to the tricuspid valve moving down during ventricular systole

○   E   reflects opening of the tricuspid valve and fall in right atrial pressure

71   **In a healthy 70 kg male at rest, the normal coronary blood flow is**

○   A   100 mL/min

○   B   250 mL/min

○   C   500 mL/min

○   D   750 mL/min

○   E   1000 mL/min

72 The superficial radial nerve

○ A runs between the brachioradialis and extensor carpi radialis longus

○ B runs between the brachialis and brachioradialis

○ C is at a high risk of injury during the posterior approach to the forearm

○ D supplies most of the muscles in the posterior compartment of the forearm

○ E is difficult to see during surgery

73 In achondroplasia, clinical features include the following EXCEPT

○ A excessive lordosis

○ B trident hands

○ C small nasal bridges

○ D hypotonia during the first year of life

○ E short trunk

74 The most common problem following total knee replacement involves

○ A infection

○ B incorrect prosthesis size

○ C chronic pain

○ D cosmesis

○ E patellar tracking

75 During the lateral (Hardinge's) approach to the hip, which of the following nerves can be injured?

○ A tibial

○ B sciatic

○ C inferior gluteal

○ D superior gluteal

○ E obturator

76 A 68-year-old man develops a massive acute myocardial infarction and dies in hospital while being resuscitated in the Emergency Department. An autopsy is performed and, while you are inspecting the heart, you note that it has undergone necrosis as expected. Which type of necrosis is found to be consistent with the pathology of this disease?

○ A coagulative necrosis

○ B liquefactive necrosis

○ C fat necrosis

○ D fibrinoid necrosis

○ E caseating necrosis

77 Which one of the following laboratory stains is used to identify amyloid staining in pathological tissue sections?

○ A Prussian blue

○ B Congo red

○ C haematoxylin & eosin

○ D oil red-O

○ E periodic acid–Schiff (PAS)

78   Diagnostic specificity is defined as

- ○   A   probability of a negative diagnostic test in the presence of disease
- ○   B   probability of a positive diagnostic test in the presence of disease
- ○   C   probability of a negative diagnostic test in the absence of disease
- ○   D   probability of a positive diagnostic test in the absence of disease
- ○   E   probability of being disease-free and test-negative within all people testing negative

79   Sertoli cells

- ○   A   are involved in the nurturing of sperm cells within the seminiferous tubules
- ○   B   synthesise testosterone
- ○   C   secrete testosterone in response to LH
- ○   D   are known as interstitial cells of the testes
- ○   E   are able to continue proliferating once fully differentiated

80   In the induction of anaesthesia

- ○   A   thiopentone injection results in a delayed recovery owing to its high lipid solubility
- ○   B   propofol commonly causes nausea on recovery
- ○   C   ketamine is a stimulant that works by dissociation
- ○   D   ketamine is routinely used in adult anaesthesia
- ○   E   ketamine may cause a bradycardia on injection

81   Which of the following is the strongest of all the other risk factors in the development of gastric carcinoma?

- ○   A   *Helicobacter pylori*
- ○   B   atrophic gastritis
- ○   C   blood group A
- ○   D   pernicious anaemia
- ○   E   low socioeconomic class

82   The first step in the management of an episode of massive haemetemesis is

- ○   A   insertion of two large bore IV cannulae
- ○   B   urgent endoscopy
- ○   C   urgent angiography
- ○   D   clearing and securing the airway
- ○   E   resuscitation with fluids and blood products

83   All of the following statements regarding prostate cancer are true EXCEPT

- ○   A   it is the 2nd leading cause of male cancer deaths
- ○   B   the lifetime risk of microscopic prostate cancer in all men is 30%
- ○   C   the incidence is decreasing due to screening measures
- ○   D   the lifetime risk of developing overt disease is 10%
- ○   E   consumption of carrots and cereals may have some protective effect

84   **All of the following statements regarding polytetrafluoroethylene (polytef or PTFE) are correct EXCEPT**

○   A   pre-clotting is not required before use

○   B   it allows tissue ingrowth and neointima formation

○   C   it is a hydrophobic non-elastic polymer

○   D   platelet deposition may occur on its surface

○   E   it is used in the creation of AV fistulae

85   **All of the following drugs may cause acute pancreatitis EXCEPT**

○   A   frusemide

○   B   azathioprine

○   C   didanosine

○   D   tetracycline

○   E   omeprazole

86   **The operation of choice for treatment of a strangulated femoral hernia, which may most likely contain infracted small bowel, is**

○   A   McEvedy's abdominal approach

○   B   Lothiessen's high approach

○   C   Lockwood's crural or low approach

○   D   Bassini's low repair

○   E   lower midline laparotomy

87   A Richter's hernia refers to a hernia that

○   A   contains two loops of small bowel within it

○   B   contains a perforated appendix

○   C   contains part of the wall of the bowel

○   D   protrudes through the linea semilunaris

○   E   causes intestinal obstruction commonly

88   The classical visual field defect caused by a pituitary adenoma will be a

○   A   homonymous hemianopia

○   B   bitemporal hemianopia

○   C   bitemporal inferior quadrantanopia

○   D   binasal hemianopia

○   E   unilateral visual loss

89   All of the following statements about 5-FU are correct EXCEPT

○   A   it is indicated in the adjuvant treatment of rectal cancers

○   B   it interferes with DNA synthesis by reducing the availability of thymidylic acid

○   C   it is used in the treatment of solid cancers

○   D   it is an alkylating agent

○   E   it inhibits pyrimidine rather than purine synthesis

90 **Which of the following anticancer drugs would be classified as an alkylating agent?**

- [ ] A doxorubicin
- [ ] B methotrexate
- [ ] C cytarabine
- [ ] D vincristine
- [ ] E cisplatin

PRACTICE PAPER 3: ANSWERS AND TEACHING NOTES

PRACTICE PAPER 3: ANSWERS AND TEACHING NOTES

1   B

L4 dermatome supplies the sensation of the medial leg from the knee down to the medial aspect of the big toe. L3 primarily supplies the superior knee and medial thigh region. L5 supplies the lateral leg and S1 the lateral foot and heel.

2   D

Quadratus femoris is a lateral rotator of the hip joint as it connects the lateral border of the ischial tuberosity to the quadrate tubercle of the femur. All the others listed abduct the hip joint acting together.

3   C

Meralgia paraesthetica refers to compression of the lateral femoral cutaneous nerve as it passes through or just under the inguinal ligament just medial to the anterior superior iliac spine. Compression of the nerve results in symptoms in the anteromedial thigh region.

4   C

The small cardiac vein accompanies the marginal artery along the inferior aspect of the heart and drains into the coronary sinus near its termination. The great cardiac vein accompanies the left anterior descending artery and the middle cardiac vein with the posterior interventricular artery.

5 E

Pain arising from the heart travels within visceral afferent nerve fibres, which can run within the upper thoracic splanchnic nerves to reach the sympathetic chain, or within the middle and inferior cardiac cervical nerves to reach the sympathetic chain and then further onto T1–T2 levels.

6 D

The thoracic duct drains everything below the level of the diaphragm as well as all structures on the left hand side of the body above the diaphragm.

7 A

The dorsal primary rami supply the deep muscles of the back such as erector spinae. Rami communicantes are involved in autonomic communications and are classed as grey (unmyelinated) or white (myelinated). Ventral rami supply all other muscles anteriorly and make up the remaining nerve root plexuses.

8 B

The following nerves provide the afferent limb of the corresponding reflexes:

- ophthalmic division of the trigeminal – blink reflex
- maxillary division of the trigeminal – sneeze reflex
- mandibular division of the trigeminal – jaw jerk
- glossopharyngeal nerve – gag reflex
- vagus nerve – cough reflex

9   D

The pterygopalatine fossa communicates with the mouth, nose, eyes and middle cranial fossa through many foramina directly. The maxillary sinus communicates via the nose through the middle meatus so any connection to the pterygopalatine fossa is indirect.

10   E

The abducent nerve runs into the medial wall of the cavernous sinus running immediately lateral to the internal carotid artery before passing into the orbit through the superior orbital fissure. All the other nerves run in the lateral wall of the cavernous sinus.

11   C

The central medullary chemoreceptors are sensitive to changes in pCO_2 via changes in H^+ (pH). The peripheral chemoreceptors located in the carotid and aortic bodies are sensitive to hypercapnia, hypoxaemia, as well as acidaemia, and hyperkalaemia. The glomus cell (type I) is responsible for sensing these changes and appropriate feedback via the IX and X cranial nerves.

12   A

The pudendal nerve block can be useful in performing episiotomies. The pudendal nerve also supplies the external anal sphincters thus rendering loss of faecal continence if it is anaesthetised. The inferior gluteal nerve supplies the gluteus maximus muscle and the superior gluteal nerve is motor supply to the gluteus medius and minimus as well as tensor fasciae latae. The ventral rami of S3 and S4 are involved in supplying the levator ani muscle, which also contributes to the mechanism of continence, but in a more physiological mechanism via the puborectalis sling.

13 D

Lateral umbilical folds – inferior epigastric arteries

Medial umbilical folds – obliterated umbilical arteries

Median umbilical fold – caudal remnant of ventral mesentery containing urachus

14 D

The gastroduodenal artery classically passes behind the first part of the duodenum (D1). Posterior ulcers that perforate through the wall of the duodenum may erode into this artery resulting in life-threatening haemorrhage.

15 D

Pronephros – develops in 3rd week but never develops fully

Mesonephric ducts – develop in males to form vas deferens and epididymis; also known as the Wolffian ducts

Metanephric ducts – develop into the ureter, pelvis, calyces and collecting tubule

Paramesonephric ducts – rise parallel to mesonephric ducts to form the uterus and uterine tubes

16   E

The foramina of Magendie (midline) and Luschka (lateral) in the roof of the 4th ventricle communicate directly into the subarachnoid space. The interventricular foramen of Munro connects the two lateral ventricles together. CSF is produced by the choroid plexus and absorbed by the arachnoid granulations (villi) to return to the venous system.

17   B

Malignant hyperpyrexia is an autosomal dominant condition with an incidence of 1:200,000. It produces a hypermetabolic state of skeletal muscle on exposure to general anaesthetics or muscle relaxants, which produces hyperthermia as a side effect. Muscle rigidity and rhabdomyolysis can occur with resulting hyperkalaemia and multi-organ failure. Treatment is supportive with IV fluids, dantrolene sodium, cooling, forced diuresis and intensive care as necessary.

18   C

Mycophenolate inhibits enzymes in the pathway of purine synthesis and is more effective and selective than azathioprine in preventing acute rejection episodes in transplanted organs. It blocks proliferation of T and B cells, thereby inhibiting formation of antibodies and generation of cytotoxic T cells.

19   D

Exotoxins are secreted by both Gram-positive and Gram-negative bacteria whereas endotoxins are found within cell walls of Gram-negative bacteria only. The main defence against these secreted toxins are antibodies such as IgG and IgM. A clinical example of this is the tetanus toxin and the tetanus immunoglobulin injected to help counter its effects.

20 E

Interferons are a heterogeneous group of endogenous glycoproteins, which inhibit the growth of viruses, bacteria, protozoa and cancer cells by blocking the translation of proteins. They are the most important part of the non-specific defence response to viral infections. Interferons classically appear within hours of initiation of viral replication in contrast to antibodies, which take some days to appear. They are species specific so therapy from animal interferons is ineffective in humans.

21 D

Hepatitis B is a dsDNA virus which belongs to the Hepadnaviridae group. Transmission occurs via three main routes: blood inoculation, sexual transmission, or vertically through childbirth or breastfeeding. The risk of HIV transmission following needlestick injury is 0.3% and HBV is 3% approximately. The HBV vaccine is a recombinant DNA vaccine.

22 B

Bacteroides organisms are anaerobic, non-spore forming, Gram-negative rods normally found within the human colon. They can cause endogenous infections and lead to peritonitis, sepsis and abscess formation. The polysaccharide capsule of the Bacteroides group is responsible for the high virulence factor. Shigella, salmonella, and vibrio are all enteric pathogens that cause gastroenteritis. *Helicobacter pylori* is a well-known cause of gastritis and is limited to the upper GI tract.

23   D

Numerous reasons exist for splenectomy in the non-trauma setting. The incidence of elective splenectomy in the UK has declined as this was used in the staging of lymphomas previously. Any cause of hypersplenism or thrombocytopenia resulting from hypersplenism can justify a splenectomy, as very large spleens can be symptomatic as well as have a very high incidence of rupture from trauma. Spleens occasionally may cause pressure symptoms if large enough.

24   A

The asplenic patient is at risk of infections from encapsulated organisms such as streptococci, *Neisseria meningitides, Haemophilus influenza*. The commonest infection to affect the asplenic patient out of this group is *Streptococcus pneumoniae*. Regular immunisations as well as penicillin prophylaxis is mandatory for these patients.

25   A

Neurogenic shock is that caused by the sudden loss of the sympathetic nervous system signals to the smooth muscle in vessel walls. This results in the triad of bradycardia, hypotension and peripheral vasodilation resulting from loss of sympathetic tone. This should be distinguished from septic shock, which results classically in a tachycardia and hypotension.

26   D

Sudden cessation in smoking causes a rebound tachycardia and hypertension, which is temporary and mostly resultant from the irritability and depression of cravings. Cardiovascular and respiratory function will improve long term and aid in recovery from surgery, anaesthesia and wound healing on stopping smoking. Effects are related to the volume and frequency of smoking for individual patients.

27   E

All CVP lines and Swan–Ganz catheters should be inserted under the strictest of aseptic technique, as infection is the commonest complication of these procedures.

28   C

Suxamethonium is a short-acting, depolarising muscle relaxant useful in anaesthesia for performing intubation in the induction phase. It is structurally similar to the ACh molecule (double ACh structure) and has a very short half-life of a few minutes, and complete metabolism by plasma cholinesterase in 5–10 minutes.

29   A

Ascites formation in cirrhosis is due to disruption of Starling's forces within the abdominal circulation. The low protein (albumin) allows for a low oncotic pressure of fluid drawback into the portal circulation from the interstitial spaces and the venous hypertension also forces the outward hydrostatic pressure equally contributing to ascitic formation. Spironolactone is useful in the treatment of ascites due to liver cirrhosis. This drug antagonises the effects of aldosterone, which is found in very high levels within the plasma due to its lack of metabolism in the cirrhotic liver.

30   D

Acid is secreted from the parietal cells within the stomach under neurohormonal influence. The highest concentration of these cells within the stomach are found in the gastric antrum. Evidence-based research also reveals that the pyloric antrum is the commonest location for *Helicobacter pylori* within the stomach and it is this location that is always biopsied in searching for *Helicobacter pylori*.

31   D

Sick euthyroid syndrome consists of abnormalities in markers of thyroid function resulting from any acute illness without actually affecting thyroid function. The following changes may occur in a clinical euthyroid patient:

- decreased binding proteins and affinity of binding proteins
- decreased TSH
- decreased peripheral conversion of T_4 to T_3

32   D

High protein diets should be avoided in chronic renal failure as this increases the urea load on the kidney. Severe protein restriction is also not advised, especially in haemodialysis, as more protein is lost through filtration. A balanced protein intake is required at about 0.5 g/kg/day in chronic renal failure.

33   D

Pancoast's tumour of the apex of the lung may produce an ipsilateral Horner's syndrome, which results in the signs of meiosis, enophthalmos, ptosis and anhidrosis of the side of the face.

34   B

Supracondylar fractures of the femur jeopardise the popliteal neurovascular bundle, in particular the popliteal artery. The sciatic nerve divides into its two terminal branches above the popliteal fossa, and the deep femoral artery has only a few geniculate branches participating around the knee. The long and short saphenous veins are subcutaneous veins lying medial to the knee or inferior to the popliteal fossa respectively.

35   A

The posterior interosseous nerve is the terminal motor branch of the radial nerve and supplies the extensor muscles from the common extensor origin distally. The brachioradialis and extensor carpi radialis longus muscles are directly supplied by the radial nerve and arise from the upper two-thirds and lower one-third of the lateral supracondylar ridge of the humerus, respectively.

36   A

The triquetral bone participates in the ulnocarpal joint and articulates with the triangular articular disc proximally. The pisiform bone is related anteromedially and hamate bone distally. During forced hyperextension of the wrist joint, anterior dislocation of the lunate bone can cause a carpal tunnel syndrome.

37   E

This patient has undergone an internal fixation of the tibia following a fracture. He is at very high risk of a compartment syndrome in that leg. He may very likely have a compartment syndrome, but that may also be caused by a tight cast amongst the causes already listed such as fractures and surgery. The first step in this case is to split the plaster cast and dressing and relieve any pressure as well as elevate the leg and prescribe analgesia. This should resolve most of his symptoms; however, if shortly after he continues to have signs and symptoms, then compartment syndrome should be suspected. Urgent senior review with fasciotomies in theatres is the next step. Compartment pressure monitoring is an adjunct to the clinical scenario here.

38   B

Drainage of the right testicular vein normally occurs into the inferior vena cava and the left testicular vein into the left renal vein. Both testicular arteries arise from the abdominal aorta and hence lymphatic drainage is to the para-aortic nodes.

39   D

CHARGE association is a sporadic condition associated with multiple congenital anomalies: C, coloboma (failure of eyeball closure) and cranial nerve palsies (facial nerve); H, heart disease; A, atresia choanae; R, retarded growth; G, genital abnormalities; E, ear abnormalities and deafness. Patients may also have laryngotracheal abnormalities.

40   E

Predisposing factors can be divided into local or general, the commonest causes being nasal. Any condition leading to blockage of the sinus ostia may lead to secretion retention and predisposition towards infection. Local causes can be due to upper respiratory tract infections, rhinitis, nasal polyps, tumours and foreign bodies, nasal anatomical variations, dental problems, swimming and diving and sinus fractures. General causes are debilitation, immuno-compromisation, mucociliary disorders (Kartagener's syndrome, cystic fibrosis) and atmospheric pollutants (dust, fumes).

41   D

Complications can be divided into immediate, intermediate and late.

- **Immediate**: anaesthetic, damage to local structures (cricoid cartilage, recurrent laryngeal nerve, oesophagus, brachiocephalic vein, thyroid – not enough to cause hypothyroidism, mostly bleeding), cardiac arrest and primary haemorrhage.

- **Intermediate**: displacement of tube, surgical emphysema, pneumothorax, obstruction of tube, infection and tracheal necrosis.

- **Late**: bubglottic/tracheal stenosis, decannulation difficulty, tracheocutaneous fistula and scar (hypertrophic, keloid).

42   B

90% of malignant oral cavity tumours are squamous cell carcinomas accounting for <2% of malignancies in the UK. The commonest site is the lateral border of the tongue, presenting as an ulcer or an exophytic lesion. Aetiological factors include smoking and chewing tobacco, and high alcohol consumption. The tonsils and soft palate are actually within the oropharynx, not the oral cavity.

43   E

The commonest cause of fever 1-day post upper GI surgery is atelectasis from retained secretions in the small bronchi. UTIs are catheter related usually and take a few days to develop rather than in the immediate postoperative period. Pulmonary emboli develop from deep vein thromboses, which also take a few days to develop. Anastomotic leaks are classically seen from day 5 onwards as are wound infections.

44   C

Verres needles are designed to be inserted under blind vision to establish a pneumoperitoneum. Most surgeons do not recommend their use as it is a blind procedure and damage to viscera can occur with a modest risk. When employing the open (Hasson's) approach, the dissection into the peritoneum is much safer, as it is done under direct vision.

45   D

The blood supply to the oesophagus is classically divided into thirds. The upper third is supplied by branches of the inferior thyroid artery, the middle third from aortic oesophageal branches, and the lower third mainly from the left gastric artery, although contributions from the inferior phrenic are also received. The pericardiophrenic arterial branch of the internal thoracic acts as the superior diaphragmatic supply, but does not contribute branches to the oesophagus.

46   C

High anal fistulae can be difficult to manage as their treatment can involve dividing the anal sphincters. A loose seton helps establish drainage of sepsis, which is of great importance as the first step in managing any anal fistula. High fistulae are seen in Crohn's disease rather than ulcerative colitis.

47   E

Extraintestinal manifestations of ulcerative colitis include ankylosing spondylitis, arthritis, uveitis, pyoderma gangrenosum, erythema nodosum and sclerosing cholangitis. Smoking unusually appears to be protective against the development of UC.

48   C

Femoral hernias occur through the femoral canal, which is under the inguinal ligament, just medial to the femoral vein. These hernias present as a lump in the groin situated below and lateral to the pubic tubercle, often as an emergency, and more commonly in elderly women. Inguinal hernias present as a lump in the groin just above and medial to the pubic tubercle.

49   A

Proximal stomas, such as jejunostomies for example, are associated with very high outputs owing to the increased secretions from the GI tract and pancreaticobiliary enzymes. The more distal position allows these fluids, along with most of the oral intake, to be digested and absorbed to a greater degree and hence less stoma output. Proximal stomas can be associated with dehydration, electrolyte abnormalities and renal failure.

50   E

Any cause of shock may result in metabolic acidosis as the inadequate perfusion results in an anaerobic metabolic response in addition to the production of lactate. Persistent vomiting typically results in a large loss of gastric acid and hence, a metabolic alkalosis.

51   E

The thoracodorsal nerve supplies the latissimus dorsi muscle, which is one of the major adductors of the shoulder joint as well as an extensor and medial rotator. A winged scapula would result from an injury to the long thoracic nerve of Bell, which arises from the roots of C5, 6 and 7 of the brachial plexus. Both of these nerves are commonly encountered in axillary dissection procedures and can be injured here as well.

52   A

Diverticular disease occurs in the colon more frequently in the developed countries and increases with increasing age. It is not inherited and has no known risk of causing colorectal cancers. There are theories suggesting that their development may be due to high intraluminal pressures arising from diets that lack fibre and cause the colon to strain in propelling the stools along. Diverticular disease may present as diverticulitis, although it may also present as obstruction, perforation, or even as a fistula into surrounding organs such as bladder, uterus, vagina and even skin.

53   E

The deep ring of the inguinal canal is a defect in the transversalis fascia and is situated 2 cm above the midpoint of the inguinal ligament. It has the inferior epigastric artery on its medial aspect and it is this structure that is used to define Hasselbach's triangle. Indirect inguinal hernias pass through the deep ring and are lateral to this vessel. Direct hernias in contrast, pass through the posterior wall, medial to the inferior epigastric artery.

54   A

Parastomal hernias spread and stretch the tissue planes making stoma closure technically easier than a normal stoma. Upon reversal of the stoma, the hernia repair can be undertaken at the same operation.

55   A

Volume depletion is not likely as the patient did not complain of diarrhoea and vomiting. The ultrasound scan would have excluded ureteric stenosis (hydronephrosis) and transplanted renal artery stenosis. Residual acute tubular necrosis does not usually lead to a jump in the serum creatinine level. The serum creatinine levels tend to plateau at a level above the normal range in such a case. Acute rejection should be suspected in this case and can be proven on an urgent biopsy.

56   B

Hiatus hernia is a protrusion of a viscus, usually stomach or upper oesophagus, through the oesophageal hiatus. They are usually classed as being of the sliding or rolling variety and may even result in strangulation or perforation; however, obstruction does not typically occur from these hernias.

57   C

The management of a pregnant woman in the trauma setting is no different from that of a normal patient. In this case the mother rather than the fetus takes priority and an obstetrician needs to be involved from early on. A special consideration that needs to be addressed is that, in mid to late pregnancy, a large uterus may compress the IVC when lying in the supine position, and hence a left lateral position whenever possible will provide a better volume return to the heart, as there is lack of caval compression. Pregnant women exhibit slightly altered physiology, which needs to be considered as well; they may not show signs of haemorrhage as they have a larger vascular volume within them.

58   C

Flexion–distraction spinal injuries do not involve the limbs unless part of a multi-trauma case. Any injury or treatment to a limb in which muscles may become oedematous within a tight fascial compartment will lead to compartment syndrome. Isolated spinal injuries would not result in such a syndrome.

59   D

Intraosseous needle insertion is not without its recognised complications. Musculocutaneous fistulae are not recognised complications as they do not exist. A fistula is an abnormal communication between two epithelial surfaces and an abscess or infection may drain from the muscle into the skin; however, this would by definition not be called a musculocutaneous fistula.

60   C

	Vol of blood loss	% blood loss
Class I	<750 mL	up to 15%
Class II	750–1500 mL	15–30%
Class III	1500–2000 mL	30–40%
Class IV	>2000 mL	>40%

61   A

Spontaneous secondary pneumothoraces occur secondary to lung pathology such as cancer, infection, or airways disease. Marfan's syndrome results in a primary (unknown) pneumothorax.

62   E

Dead space is the volume of air that has to be ventilated, but does not actually take part in gas exchange. Anatomical dead space is the volume that does not mix with air in the alveoli, and physiological dead space is the volume of air that may reach the alveoli, but does not take part in gas exchange, eg owing to lack of perfusion. Anatomical dead space will be increased in the standing position, with larger lung volumes and bronchodilation. Physiological dead space is increased in hypotension, hypoventilation, pulmonary embolus, emphysema and positive pressure ventilation.

63   A

Cushing's syndrome classically causes a hypokalaemia and metabolic alkalosis resulting in a high bicarbonate serum level and positive base excess. Starvation and septicaemia will both result in metabolic acidosis, the respiratory disorders with a respiratory acidosis in myasthenia gravis owing to hypoventilation, and respiratory alkalosis in pulmonary embolus owing to hyperventilation and tachypnoea.

64   C

Causes of fever include, but are not limited to: illness, exercise, heatstroke, hyperthyroidism, malignant hyperpyrexia, failure of the heat-loss mechanism (dehydration), and by anterior hypothalamic lesions (neoplasia, ischaemia, surgery).

65   E

ARDS is an acute syndrome characterised by respiratory failure with the formation of non-cardiogenic pulmonary oedema, leading to reduced lung compliance and hypoxaemia refractory to oxygen therapy. The pulmonary wedge pressure is <16 mmHg. Diffuse pulmonary infiltrates are seen and the PO_2/FiO2 ratio is <26.6 kPa (200 mmHg).

66   B

Physiological changes resulting from a large pulmonary embolus include:

- increased pulmonary vascular resistance
- pulmonary hypertension
- decreased left ventricular output
- increased right ventricular afterload
- decreased lung compliance
- impaired gas exchange

67   C

Drugs that interact with grapefruit and/or grapefruit juice undergo cytochrome p450 oxidative metabolism in the intestinal wall or liver. Grapefruit juice contains various furanocoumarins, which have been demonstrated to affect the cytochrome p450 system, especially at the isoenzyme CYP3A4. From the immunosuppressive agents, both cyclosporine and tacrolimus may have reduced metabolism from consumption of grapefruit juice leading to toxic effects.

68   D

A gay patient who has been in a long and stable relationship can be an organ donor; he is probably of a lower risk group than say a young promiscuous heterosexual. Organ donation after cardiac death from withdrawal of treatment is permissible. The patient is not necessarily too old to be a donor. It depends on what other comorbidities are present. If he is a diabetic and/or has long-standing hypertension and, at retrieval, the renal arteries show signs of heavy deposition of atheroma, then one is minded to turn down the kidneys for transplantation.

69   D

Correct phases of the cardiac action potential of ventricular muscles cell are:

Phase 0 – initial rapid depolarisation

Phase 1 – rapid repolarisation

Phase 2 – slow repolarisation plateau

Phase 3 – rapid repolarisation

Phase 4 – resting membrane potential

70   D

- a wave – prominent in atrial systole
- c wave – synchronous with the carotid pulse wave
- v wave – reflects a rise in atrial pressure before the tricuspid valve opens
- x descent – due to the tricuspid valve moving down during ventricular systole
- y descent – reflects opening of tricuspid valve and fall in right atrial pressure

71   B

The normal coronary blood flow to the heart is 250 mL/min in the average 70 kg healthy young male adult at rest. This can rise to 1 L/m on exercise.

72   A

The radial nerve enters the forearm anterior to the lateral epicondyle, runs between the brachialis and brachioradialis and divides into the superficial radial and posterior interosseous nerve (PIN). The PIN splits the supinator (site of damage during retraction of the muscle) and supplies all of the extensor muscles except the brachioradialis, extensor carpi radialis brevis and extensor carpi radialis longus. The superficial radial nerve passes to the dorsal radial surface of the hand in the distal third of the forearm by passing between the brachioradialis and extensor carpi radialis longus. It can be visualised during the anterior approach to the forearm.

73   E

Clinical features of achondroplasia include small nasal bridges, button noses, trident hands (inability to approximate extended middle and ring fingers), lumbar stenosis, excessive lordosis, hypotonia during the first year of life, radial head subluxation, frontal bossing and a normal trunk but short limbs (rhizomelic).

74   E

The technical goals of a knee replacement are (1) restoration of mechanical alignment; (2) preservation of joint line; (3) balanced ligaments; and (4) maintenance of the Q angle (the angle formed by the intersection of the extensor mechanism axis above the patella, with the axis of the patella tendon). To avoid lateral subluxation of the patella the femoral component is positioned laterally and rotated externally; internal rotation of the tibial component is avoided; the patellar component is medialised, and the joint position is maintained.

75   D

In the lateral approach, the skin and the fascia lata are incised to expose the gluteus medius and the vastus lateralis muscles. The gluteus medius is incised from the greater trochanter, leaving a cuff of tissue. This incision is extended to split the gluteus medius proximally, and distally the vastus is split along its anterior part down to the femoral shaft. The gluteus minimus is detached from its insertion and the hip is exposed after incising the joint capsule. The superior gluteal nerve can be damaged (and the gluteus medius denervated) if the gluteus medius is split >5 cm proximal to the greater trochanter.

76   A

Coagulative necrosis commonly occurs in fibrous or muscular tissue where the outline of the cell is retained, but not the cell nucleus. The brain undergoes liquefactive necrosis classically, which results from complete hydrolysis of the cell. Caseating necrosis is seen in cases of TB and may represent a combination of coagulative and liquefactive necrosis. Fat necrosis usually occurs in abdominal wall, pancreatic or breast tissue that has sustained trauma and has been damaged by lipases. Fibrinoid necrosis may be seen in damaged vessel walls where plasma proteins accumulate.

77   B

Congo red stains are used to identify and stain tissues containing amyloid. When polarised light is used, the amyloid is identified by its apple-green birefringence.

78   C

Specificity refers to how well a test picks up disease-free individuals. It is expressed as a proportion of those disease-free individuals testing negative (true negatives) out of all disease-free individuals (true negatives plus false positives).

79   A

Sertoli cells are regarded as 'mother cells' providing nutrition and well-being to the sperm cells within the seminiferous tubules. Once differentiated, they stop proliferating. Leydig cells or interstitial cells synthesise and secrete testosterone in response to hormonal stimulation by LH and FSH.

80   C

Ketamine is a stimulant that works by dissociation. It commonly causes a tachycardia and rise in blood pressure on injection. Its use is commonly within paediatric anaesthesia. The commonest side effects are nightmares and hallucinations.

81   B

Atrophic gastritis and hypogammaglobulinaemia are both associated with a 30-fold increase in risk of developing gastric carcinoma. The other conditions listed have proven risks but are not as great.

82   D

Airway, breathing and circulation in that order are always the mainstay of any resuscitation measures. Massive haematemesis requires resuscitation first; then proceed or transfer to definitive treatment.

83   C

The incidence of prostate cancer is rising as the general elderly population increases. The average age of death in men is rising and hence prostate cancer will be more prevalent.

84   D

The smooth inert surface of PTFE as well as the negatively charged surface inhibits platelet deposition. Bleeding can sometimes be a problem through pores made by suture needles.

85 E

H_2 antagonists such as cimetidine and ranitidine can lead to pancreatitis but not proton pump inhibitors.

86 A

The abdominal approach is best reserved where bowel resection is contemplated. An inguinal or high approach is used to repair co-existing inguinal hernias or where the diagnosis is in doubt. For small uncomplicated femoral hernias in the elective setting, the low or crural approach is preferable.

87 C

Richter's hernia contains only part of the bowel wall within it and hence do not classically cause an obstruction. Amyand's hernia contains a perforated appendix within an inguinal hernia. A hernia through the linea semilunaris is called a Spigelian hernia. Maydl's hernia contains loops of small bowel often forming a W-shaped configuration.

88 B

The central location of the pituitary gland within the sella turcica causes compression of the medial aspects of the optic chiasm. The resultant visual field defect is bitemporal hemianopia.

89   D

5-FU is commonly used in the treatment of colorectal cancers. It belongs to the group of antimetabolites and inhibits DNA synthesis accordingly by interfering with pyrimidine synthesis.

90   E

Cisplatin along with busulphan, chlorambucil, chlormethine and cyclophosphamide are some of the drugs classed as alkylating agents. Doxorubicin is an antibiotic, vincristine is a vinca alkaloid, methotrexate is an antimetabolite, and cytarabine inhibits DNA polymerase.

PRACTICE PAPER 4: QUESTIONS

PRACTICE PAPER 4: QUESTIONS

1 Calot's triangle

- ○ A is bounded laterally by the common hepatic duct
- ○ B is bounded medially by the right hepatic duct
- ○ C is bounded laterally by the cystic duct
- ○ D contains the left hepatic duct
- ○ E contains the hepatic artery

2 The epiploic foramen

- ○ A is the opening of the lesser sac on the left side of the abdomen
- ○ B lies anterior to the superior vena cava
- ○ C lies inferior to the quadrate lobe of the liver
- ○ D is superior to the third part of the duodenum
- ○ E contains the hepatic artery lying on the left of the common bile duct in the anterior border

3 The transpyloric plane of Addison

- ○ A passes through the inferior border of L2
- ○ B encompasses the tail of the pancreas
- ○ C is at the same level as the 8th costal cartilages
- ○ D the inferior mesenteric artery commences at this level
- ○ E lies halfway between the jugular notch and pubic symphysis

4 **Which of the following statement is true regarding the planes of the abdomen**

- [ ] A the subcostal plane runs through the inferior border of L3
- [ ] B the transtubercular plane runs through the body of L5
- [ ] C the sagittal planes run through the midpoint of the inguinal ligament
- [ ] D the transpyloric plane runs through the superior border of L2
- [ ] E the transumbilical plane runs through the L2/3 intervertebral disc

5 **Which of the following statement is true regarding the adrenal glands**

- [ ] A the right adrenal is more medial than the left
- [ ] B the right adrenal lies lateral to the superior phrenic vessels
- [ ] C the left adrenal lies posterior to the splenic artery
- [ ] D the right adrenal vein drains into the right renal vein
- [ ] E cortisol is secreted by the zona glomerulosa

6 **Which of the following statement is true regarding the pharyngeal arches and pouches**

- [ ] A the superior parathyroid glands are derived from the 4th pharyngeal pouch
- [ ] B the mandible is derived from the 2nd pharyngeal arch
- [ ] C the 3rd pharyngeal arch is supplied by the vagus nerve
- [ ] D the pharyngeal arches consist of endoderm and ectoderm only
- [ ] E the inferior parathyroid glands are derived from the 5th pharyngeal pouch

7   The facial nerve passes through

- ○ A   the superior orbital fissure
- ○ B   the foramen ovale
- ○ C   the foramen rotundum
- ○ D   the stylomastoid foramen
- ○ E   the petrosquamous fissure

8   Extensor compartment II of the wrist contains

- ○ A   abductor pollicis longus
- ○ B   extensor pollicis brevis
- ○ C   extensor carpi radialis
- ○ D   extensor pollicis longus
- ○ E   extensor digitorum

9   The quadrilateral space

- ○ A   is bounded inferiorly by teres minor
- ○ B   is bounded inferiorly by subscapularis
- ○ C   is bounded laterally by the long head of triceps
- ○ D   is bounded inferiorly by teres major
- ○ E   contains the radial nerve

10 **The carpal tunnel does NOT contain**

○ A flexor digitorum superficialis

○ B flexor digitorum profundus

○ C median nerve

○ D flexor pollicis longus

○ E flexor carpi ulnaris

11 **Which statement is true of the brachial plexus?**

○ A the medial cord continues as the musculocutaneous nerve

○ B the posterior cord continues as the axillary nerve

○ C the lateral cord continues as the axillary nerve

○ D the nerve to subclavius is a branch of the C8 nerve root

○ E the suprascapular nerve is a branch of the lower trunk

12 **Which statement is true of diaphragmatic openings?**

○ A the thoracic duct passes through the opening at T12

○ B the aorta passes through the opening at T10

○ C the left phrenic nerve passes through the opening at T8

○ D the right gastric artery passes through the opening at T10

○ E the azygous vein passes through the opening at T10

13 Structures NOT at risk of being damaged during carotid endarterectomy include the

○ A hypoglossal nerve

○ B greater auricular nerve

○ C vagus nerve

○ D recurrent laryngeal nerve

○ E accessory nerve

14 The abdominal aorta lies on the

○ A left of the sympathetic trunk

○ B left of the inferior mesenteric vessels

○ C left of the azygous vein

○ D right of the cisterna chyli

○ E right of the IVC

15 The right ureter in females

○ A lies beneath the third part of the duodenum at its origin

○ B runs over the ovarian artery

○ C crosses the uterine artery

○ D is crossed by the right colic artery

○ E lies beneath the bifurcation of the iliac vessels

16 The stomach bed does NOT include the

- ○ A splenic artery
- ○ B coeliac trunk
- ○ C transverse mesocolon
- ○ D left adrenal gland
- ○ E neck of the pancreas

17 Passing through the lesser sciatic foramen are the

- ○ A inferior gluteal artery
- ○ B pudendal nerve
- ○ C posterior cutaneous nerve of the thigh
- ○ D inferior gluteal nerve
- ○ E nerve to quadratus femoris

18 Which statement is true of the compartment of the leg?

- ○ A the anterior compartment contains the superficial peroneal nerve
- ○ B the lateral compartment contains the deep peroneal nerve
- ○ C the lateral compartment contains peroneus tertius
- ○ D the deep posterior compartment contains plantaris
- ○ E the posterior compartment contains the peroneal artery

19   The brachial artery

- ⃝   A   commences at the upper border of teres major
- ⃝   B   initially lies anterior to the humerus
- ⃝   C   lies medial to the median nerve proximally
- ⃝   D   lies medial to the ulnar nerve proximally
- ⃝   E   lies lateral to biceps distally

20   The muscle divided in the Hardinge approach to the hip is the

- ⃝   A   obturator internus
- ⃝   B   piriformis
- ⃝   C   gluteus maximus
- ⃝   D   superior gemellus
- ⃝   E   vastus lateralis

21   Sites of ulnar nerve entrapment include the

- ⃝   A   arcade of Frohse
- ⃝   B   carpal tunnel
- ⃝   C   lateral triangular space
- ⃝   D   arcade of Struthers
- ⃝   E   cubital fossa

22   Which statement is true of the inguinal region?

○   A   the midpoint of the inguinal ligament lies half way between the anterior superior iliac spine and the pubic symphysis

○   B   the midinguinal point lies half way between the anterior superior iliac spine and the pubic tubercle

○   C   the deep inguinal ring lies at the midinguinal point

○   D   the femoral artery lies at the midpoint of the inguinal ligament

○   E   the femoral nerve lies half way between the anterior superior iliac spine and the pubic tubercle

23   The boundaries of the inguinal canal include

○   A   the lacunar ligament are part of the roof

○   B   the inguinal ligament as part of the roof

○   C   external oblique as part of the roof

○   D   the conjoint tendon as part of the roof

○   E   the transversalis fascia as part of the roof

24   Which of these structures does NOT pass posterior to the medial malleolus?

○   A   tibialis posterior tendon

○   B   saphenous vein

○   C   flexor digitorum longus tendon

○   D   flexor hallucis longus tendon

○   E   posterior tibial artery

25 Which of these nerves does NOT lie in the lateral wall of the cavernous sinus?

○ A   trochlear nerve

○ B   occulomotor nerve

○ C   mandibular branch of the trigeminal nerve

○ D   maxillary branch of the trigeminal nerve

○ E   ophthalmic branch of the trigeminal nerve

26 Which of the following muscles does not attach to the common flexor origin of the forearm?

○ A   pronator teres

○ B   palmaris longus

○ C   flexor carpi ulnaris

○ D   flexor carpi radialis

○ E   flexor pollicis longus

27 Structures passing through the foramen magnum do NOT include the

○ A   vagus nerve

○ B   accessory nerve

○ C   medulla

○ D   meninges

○ E   vertebral arteries

28   **Which of these statements is true regarding the femoral triangle**

⭕   A   the lateral border of sartorius forms the lateral border

⭕   B   the lateral border of adductor magnus forms the medial border

⭕   C   adductor brevis forms part of the floor

⭕   D   adductor magnus forms part of the floor

⭕   E   pectineus forms part of the floor

29   **The rectus sheath does NOT contain the**

⭕   A   rectus abdominis

⭕   B   inferior epigastric vein

⭕   C   superior epigastric artery

⭕   D   lower eight thoracic nerves

⭕   E   pyramidalis

30   **Which of these is NOT part of the medial longitudinal arch of the foot?**

⭕   A   talus

⭕   B   navicular

⭕   C   cuboid

⭕   D   calcaneus

⭕   E   medial cuneiform

31   **The plane of Louis is NOT the**

○   A   level of the aortic arch

○   B   level of the third costal cartilage

○   C   level of the lower border of T4

○   D   level of the bifurcation of the trachea

○   E   level at which the azygous vein enters the superior vena cava

32   **Which of the following regarding the duodenum is incorrect?**

○   A   the duodenum is comprised of four parts

○   B   the first part lies at the level of L1

○   C   the second part lies at the level of L2

○   D   the third part lies at the level of L3

○   E   the fourth part lies at the level of L4

33   **The sciatic nerve does NOT supply which of the following muscles?**

○   A   obturator externus

○   B   semimembranosus

○   C   superior gemellus

○   D   quadratus femoris

○   E   biceps femoris

34 The braches of the posterior cord of the brachial plexus do NOT include the

- ○ A upper subscapular nerve
- ○ B lower subscapular nerve
- ○ C axillary nerve
- ○ D musculocutaneous nerve
- ○ E thoracodorsal nerve

35 The criteria for brainstem death do NOT include

- ○ A apnoeic coma requiring ventilation
- ○ B absence of sedative medications
- ○ C absence of gag reflex
- ○ D lack of response to painful stimulus to stimuli
- ○ E normal body temperature

36 Swan–Ganz catheters CANNOT be used to directly measure

- ○ A pulmonary artery wedge pressure
- ○ B mean arterial pressure
- ○ C cardiac output
- ○ D systemic vascular resistance
- ○ E central venous pressure

37 **Which statement is correct regarding the oxygen haemoglobin transport curve?**

○ A each gram of haemoglobin binds 1 mL of oxygen when fully saturated

○ B at a PaO_2 of 40 mmHg the saturation of Hb is 50%

○ C fetal haemoglobin moves the curve to the right

○ D alkaline pH moves the curve to the right

○ E increased temperature moves the curve to the right

38 **Which statement is correct regarding carbon dioxide transport?**

○ A 10% is transported as carbaminohaemoglobin

○ B the carbaminohaemoglobin dissociation curve readily saturates

○ C 20% is transported dissolved in the plasma

○ D 50% is transported as sodium bicarbonate

○ E carbonic anhydrase catalyses the reaction of CO_2 and plasma

39 **Which statement is correct regarding cerebrospinal fluid?**

○ A the normal total volume is 250 mL

○ B it passes from the lateral to the 3rd ventricles via the foramen of Munro

○ C it is reabsorbed by the choroids plexuses

○ D the rate of production is proportional to the systemic blood pressure

○ E it passes from the 3rd to the 4th ventricles via the foramen of Magendie

40 **Which statement is correct regarding respiratory volumes?**

- ○ A   the tidal volume in males is 1000 mL
- ○ B   the inspiratory reserve volume is 2000 mL
- ○ C   the vital capacity is 2000 mL
- ○ D   the residual volume is 1900 mL
- ○ E   the total lung capacity is 4000 mL

41 **The maximum safe dose of 1% lignocaine without adrenaline for a 70 kg male is**

- ○ A   14 mL
- ○ B   21 mL
- ○ C   28 mL
- ○ D   35 mL
- ○ E   40 mL

42 **Parathyroid hormone secretion is decreased by**

- ○ A   an increase in serum phosphate
- ○ B   a decrease in free Ca^{2+}
- ○ C   a decrease in serum magnesium
- ○ D   an increase in serum potassium
- ○ E   a decrease in $1,25(OH)_2D$

43   Which statement is correct regarding secretions from the adrenal glands?

⭘   A   aldosterone is produced by the zona glomerulosa

⭘   B   progesterone is produced by the zona fasiculata

⭘   C   testosterone is produced by the zona reticulosa

⭘   D   adrenaline is produced by the zona reticulosa

⭘   E   cortisol is produced by the zona glomerulosa

44   One litre of Hartman's solution contains

⭘   A   154 mmol/L of sodium

⭘   B   5 mmol/L of glucose

⭘   C   130 mmol/L of chloride

⭘   D   10 mmol/L of calcium

⭘   E   5 mmol/L of potassium

45   Volumes of gastrointestinal secretions per day are

⭘   A   3000 mL of saliva

⭘   B   2000 mL of pancreatic juices

⭘   C   2000 mL of bile

⭘   D   3500 mL of small bowel secretions

⭘   E   1500 mL of large bowel secretions

46   Which of the following is NOT true regarding gastric secretions?

- ○   A   gastrin is produced by the G cells of the pyloric glands
- ○   B   pepsinogen is produced by the chief cells
- ○   C   mucus is produced by the surface epithelial cells
- ○   D   intrinsic factor is produced by the parietal cells
- ○   E   hydrochloric acid is produced by the chief cells

47   Which of the following are NOT normally found in bile?

- ○   A   sodium chloride
- ○   B   unconjugated bilirubin
- ○   C   cholesterol
- ○   D   water
- ○   E   bile salts

48   Which of the following factors are part of the extrinsic pathway in the coagulation cascade?

- ○   A   Factor XII
- ○   B   Factor XI
- ○   C   Factor IX
- ○   D   Factor VII
- ○   E   Factor XIII

49 Functions of the terminal ileum do NOT include

- ○ A folate reuptake
- ○ B bile salt reuptake
- ○ C vitamin B_{12} uptake
- ○ D water reabsorption
- ○ E γ-globulin uptake

50 The liver does NOT synthesise

- ○ A prothrombin
- ○ B proaccelerin
- ○ C plasminogen
- ○ D antithrombin
- ○ E fibrinogen

51 Which statement is correct regarding the Renin–angiotensin system?

- ○ A antidiuretic hormone is released from the anterior pituitary
- ○ B renin is secreted by the granular cells of the juxtaglomerular apparatus
- ○ C angiotensinogen is released into the plasma only when required
- ○ D antidiuretic hormone is produced by the anterior pituitary
- ○ E angiotensin I is converted to angiotensin II by angiotensin-converting enzyme in the liver

52   Which statement is correct regarding transport in the proximal tubule of the kidney: ?

- ○ A   sodium is passively reabsorbed
- ○ B   glucose is passively reabsorbed
- ○ C   amino acids are actively reabsorbed
- ○ D   urea is actively reabsorbed
- ○ E   potassium is secreted

53   The chemoreceptors involved in maintenance of blood pressure are

- ○ A   located in the pulmonary arteries
- ○ B   stimulated by high oxygen levels
- ○ C   stimulated by alkaline pH
- ○ D   stimulated by high carbon dioxide levels
- ○ E   stimulated by stretching of the vessel walls

54   Which of the following is NOT part of the flight or fight response?

- ○ A   constriction of blood vessels
- ○ B   constriction of the pupils
- ○ C   sweating
- ○ D   increased heart rate
- ○ E   decreased GI activity

55 **Which of the following is an anion?**

○ A sodium

○ B magnesium

○ C phosphate

○ D calcium

○ E potassium

56 **Which of the following is an accessory muscle of expiration?**

○ A sternocleidomastoid

○ B pectoralis major

○ C scalenus anterior

○ D latissimus dorsi

○ E rectus abdominis

57 **Which of the following statements is NOT true regarding vitamin B_{12}?**

○ A it is necessary for maturation of red cells

○ B it is stored in the liver

○ C intrinsic factor is required for its absorption

○ D stores can last for up to a year

○ E there is a small amount in bile

58 Which of the following is an exocrine secretion of the pancreas?

O A pancreatic polypeptide

O B somatostatin

O C trypsinogen

O D glucagon

O E insulin

59 Lung compliance is increased by

O A alveolar oedema

O B pulmonary hypertension

O C atelectasis

O D pulmonary fibrosis

O E emphysema

60 The posterior pituitary releases

O A adrenocorticotropic hormone (ACTH)

O B follicle-stimulating hormone (FSH)

O C antidiuretic hormone (ADH)

O D thyroid-stimulating hormone (TSH)

O E growth hormone (GH)

61 Which of the following is NOT the correct daily requirement for an average 70 kg male?

- A 150 mmol sodium
- B 2500 mL water
- C 70 mmol calcium
- D 70 mmol potassium
- E 70 mmol chloride

62 Causes of metabolic acidosis with a normal anion gap include

- A diarrhoea
- B diabetic ketoacidosis
- C salicylate overdose
- D renal tubular acidosis
- E lactic acidosis

63 Tumour markers for testicular cancer do NOT include

- A γ-glutamyltransferase (GGT) for seminoma and NSGCT
- B human chorionic gonadotropin (γ-HCG) for seminoma and NSGCT
- C lactate dehydrogenase (LDH) for NSGCT
- D carcinoembryogenic antigen (CEA) for NSGCT
- E α-fetoprotein for NSGCT

64   Which of the following are NOT risk factors for bladder cancer?

○   A β-naphthamine

○   B   schistosoma

○   C   catheterisation

○   D   alcohol

○   E   smoking

65   Epstein–Barr virus is known to be a carcinogen for

○   A   T-cell lymphoma

○   B   non-Hodgkin's lymphoma

○   C   leukaemia

○   D   B-cell lymphoma

○   E   hepatocellular carcinoma

66   The following viruses are NOT known to be carcinogenic

○   A   Epstein–Barr virus

○   B   hepatitis B

○   C   human immunodeficiency virus

○   D   hepatitis A

○   E   human papilloma virus

67   **Multiple endocrine neoplasia 1 (MEN 1)**

- ◯   A   has an autosomal recessive inheritance
- ◯   B   has its gene located on chromosome 10
- ◯   C   is known as Sipple's syndrome
- ◯   D   commonly includes phaeochromocytoma
- ◯   E   commonly includes hyperparathyroidism

68   **Which is NOT a common feature of MEN 2B?**

- ◯   A   medullary thyroid carcinoma
- ◯   B   multiple mucosal neuromas
- ◯   C   phaeochromocytoma
- ◯   D   marfanoid appearance
- ◯   E   gastrinoma

69   **Meckel's diverticulum**

- ◯   A   is more common in females
- ◯   B   is usually 2 cm long
- ◯   C   can contain hepatic mucosa
- ◯   D   contains only the mucosa and submucosa of the intestinal wall
- ◯   E   is a remnant of the omphalomesenteric duct

70 Which of the following is NOT true regarding malignant hyperpyrexia?

○ A   it can be caused by suxamethonium

○ B   it can be caused by isoflurane

○ C   it can be caused by nitrous oxide

○ D   it dantrolene is the treatment

○ E   it occurs in 1 in 150,000

71 Characteristic signs of acute inflammation include

○ A   dolor

○ B   palor

○ C   rubor

○ D   tumour

○ E   calor

72 Types of tumour markers do NOT include

○ A   enzymes

○ B   hormones

○ C   ectopic hormones

○ D   oncofetal antibodies

○ E   oncofetal antigens

73   Apoptosis

- ○ A   is a process which results from energy deprivation
- ○ B   is initially reversible and becomes irreversible
- ○ C   is initiated by an injury
- ○ D   causes swelling of the cell
- ○ E   results in orderly vesicle formation

74   For which of the following is blood for transfusion NOT screened?

- ○ A   EBV
- ○ B   hepatitis B
- ○ C   syphilis
- ○ D   hepatitis C
- ○ E   HIV

75   Psammoma bodies on histology are characteristic of

- ○ A   follicular thyroid carcinoma
- ○ B   anaplastic thyroid carcinoma
- ○ C   papillary thyroid carcinoma
- ○ D   medullary thyroid carcinoma
- ○ E   thyroid lymphoma

76   Which of the following is NOT a Gram-negative rod?

- ○ A   *Escherichia coli*
- ○ B   *Clostridia tetani*
- ○ C   *Proteus* species
- ○ D   *Legionella*
- ○ E   *Pseudomonas*

77   Tumours that commonly metastasise to bone do NOT include

- ○ A   breast
- ○ B   lung
- ○ C   prostate
- ○ D   adrenal
- ○ E   thyroid

78   Granulomas are NOT found in

- ○ A   TB
- ○ B   sarcoidosis
- ○ C   ulcerative colitis
- ○ D   Crohn's disease
- ○ E   leprosy

79   **Dysplasia does NOT cause**

- ○   A   increased cell growth
- ○   B   cellular atypia
- ○   C   abnormal differentiation
- ○   D   a low nuclear to cytoplasmic ratio
- ○   E   pleomorphism

80   **Risk factors for malignant melanoma include**

- ○   A   fair skin
- ○   B   family history
- ○   C   continuous sun exposure
- ○   D   xeroderma pigmentosa
- ○   E   albinism

81   **Which of the following is not a benign skin lesion?**

- ○   A   Pott's peculiar tumour
- ○   B   seborrhoeic keratosis
- ○   C   hamartoma
- ○   D   Merkel cell tumour
- ○   E   Turban tumour

82   Which of the following is NOT a nutritional factor involved in wound healing?

- A   vitamin A
- B   vitamin B$_3$
- C   vitamin B$_6$
- D   zinc
- E   copper

83   Which is correct regarding cells involved in wound healing?

- A   platelets take 1 day to appear
- B   neutrophils take 2 days to appear
- C   macrophages appear immediately
- D   fibroblasts take 3 days to appear
- E   endothelial cells take 1 day to appear

84   Which of the following statements regarding cell growth is NOT true?

- A   hypertrophy is an increase in cell size
- B   hyperplasia is an increase in cell number
- C   metaplasia is the conversion of one tissue type to another
- D   teratoma is a growth of cells originating from more than one germ cell line
- E   hamartoma is an overgrowth of cell not normally found in that tissue

85   The most common type of lung cancer is

- ○   A   squamous carcinoma
- ○   B   small cell carcinoma
- ○   C   large cell carcinoma
- ○   D   adenocarcinoma
- ○   E   adenosquamous carcinoma

86   Which statement is true of pleomorphic adenoma

- ○   A   it is the second commonest salivary gland tumour
- ○   B   it usually affects the submandibular gland
- ○   C   it is more common in females
- ○   D   it approximately 10% are bilateral
- ○   E   it is commonest in the fourth and fifth decades

87   Reed–Stenberg cells are characteristic of

- ○   A   Hodgkin's lymphoma
- ○   B   non-Hodgkin's lymphoma
- ○   C   Burkitt's lymphoma
- ○   D   B-cell lymphoma
- ○   E   T-cell lymphoma

88   Risk factors for hepatocellular carcinoma do NOT include

- ○ A   hepatitis B
- ○ B   hepatitis C
- ○ C   hepatitis E
- ○ D   aflatoxin
- ○ E   anabolic steroids

89   Local factors that affect wound healing do NOT include

- ○ A   foreign bodies
- ○ B   haematoma
- ○ C   malnutrition
- ○ D   infection
- ○ E   decreased blood supply

90   Infantile hypertrophic pyloric stenosis

- ○ A   is more common in females
- ○ B   is more common in second born and subsequent children
- ○ C   usually presents at approximately 3 months old
- ○ D   causes ametabolic acidosis
- ○ E   occurs in 31,000 live births

PRACTICE PAPER 4: ANSWERS AND TEACHING NOTES

PRACTICE PAPER 4: ANSWERS AND TEACHING NOTES

1   C

The boundaries of Calot's triangle are:

Medially – the common hepatic duct

Laterally – the cystic duct

Superiorly – the visceral surface of the liver

It contains:

- the cystic artery
- cystic lymph nodes
- the right hepatic duct
- occasionally the cystic vein

2   E

The epiploic foramen is the opening of the lesser sac on the right side of the abdomen.

The boundaries of the epiploic foramen are:

Anteriorly – the free edge of the lesser omentum, containing the common bile duct on the right, hepatic artery on the left and the portal vein posteriorly

Posteriorly – the inferior vena cava and right crus of the diaphragm

Inferiorly – the first part of the duodenum

Superiorly – the caudate lobe of the liver

3   E

The transpyloric plane of Addison lies midway between the jugular notch and the pubic symphysis at the level of the lower border of the L1 vertebra.

Structures lying at this level are the:

- pyloris of the stomach
- fundus of the gallbladder
- duodenojejunal junction
- neck of the pancreas
- hila of the kidneys
- ninth costal cartilages
- superior mesenteric artery commences
- portal vein is formed.

4   B

The subcostal plane runs through the superior border of L3.

The transtubercular plane runs through the iliac tubercles, passing through the body of L5.

The transumbilical plane runs through the umbilicus at the level of the L3/4 intervertebral disc.

The sagittal planes are continuations of the midclavicular lines, running through the midinguinal points.

The transpyloric plane runs through the inferior border of L1.

5   C

The left adrenal lies more medially than the right. The left adrenal lies posterior to the splenic artery and body of the pancreas, anterior to the left crus of the diaphragm, lateral to the coeliac ganglion and left gastric vessels, and medial to the left kidney. The right adrenal lies posterior to the right lobe of the liver and IVC, anterior to the right crus of the diaphragm, and lateral to the right inferior phrenic vessels.

The zona glomerulosa secretes aldosterone, the zona fasciculata cortisol and testosterone, and the zona reticularis oestradiol and progesterone.

6   A

The pharyngeal arches are composed of mesoderm, endoderm and ectoderm. The superior parathyroids are derived from the 4th pharyngeal pouch and the inferior parathyroids are derived from the 3rd pharyngeal pouch. The mandible, maxilla and zygoma are derived from the 1st pharyngeal arch. The 3rd pharyngeal arch is supplied by the glossopharyngeal nerve.

7   D

The facial nerve traverses the facial canal, the internal auditory meatus and the stylomastoid foramen. The superior orbital foramen contains the oculomotor, trochlear, trigeminal and abducent nerves. The trigeminal nerve passes through the foramen ovale and the foramen rotundum. The petrosquamous fissure has no contents.

8   C

The contents of the extensor compartments are:

I – Abductor pollicis longus and extensor pollicis brevis

II – Extensor carpi radialis

III – Extensor pollicis longus

IV – Extensor digitorum and extensor indicis

V – Extensor digiti minimi

VI – Extensor carpi ulnaris

9   D

The boundaries of the quadrilateral space are:

Superiorly – subscapularis

Inferiorly – teres major

Medially – long head of triceps

Laterally – medial shaft of humerus

It contains:

- axillary nerve
- posterior circumflex humeral artery and vein

10   E

The contents of the carpal tunnel are:

- median nerve
- flexor digitorum superficialis
- flexor digitorum profundus
- flexor pollicis longus
- flexor carpi radialis

11   B

The lateral cord continues as the musculocutaneous nerve.

The medial cord continues as the ulnar nerve.

The posterior cord continues as the radial nerve and the axillary nerve.

The nerve to subclavius is a branch of the C6 root.

The suprascapular nerve is a branch from the upper trunk.

12   A

The openings are:

T8 – the opening for the inferior vena cava, also passing through the right phrenic nerve

T10 – the opening for the oesophagus, also passing through the left gastric artery and vein

T12 – the opening for the aorta, also passing through the thoracic duct and azygous vein

13　E

The hypoglossal, greater auricular, vagus and recurrent laryngeal nerve are all at risk during carotid endarterectomy. The superior laryngeal and accessory nerves are not.

14　C

The aorta lies on the right of the sympathetic trunk, inferior mesenteric vessels, left crus of the diaphragm and coeliac ganglion. It lies on the left of the azygous vein, cisterna chyli, thoracic duct, IVC and right crus of the diaphragm.

15　D

The right ureter lies beneath the second part of the duodenum at its origin. It is crossed by the ovarian, uterine, right colic and ileocolic arteries. It crosses the bifurcation of the iliac arteries.

16　E

The stomach bed comprises the lesser sac of the peritoneum, left crus of the diaphragm, upper left kidney, left adrenal gland, body and tail of the pancreas, spleen, splenic artery, transverse mesocolon, aorta, coeliac trunk, coeliac ganglion and lymph nodes.

17 B

The structures that pass through the lesser sciatic foramen are the pudendal nerve, nerve to obturator internus, internal pudendal artery and tendon of obturator internus.

18 E

The anterior compartment contains the deep peroneal nerve and anterior tibial artery. The lateral compartment contains the superficial peroneal nerve and no artery. Peroneus tertius is in the anterior compartment, peroneus brevis and longus are in the lateral compartment The superficial posterior compartment contains gastrocnemius, soleus and plantaris. The posterior compartment contains the posterior tibial nerve, posterior tibial artery and peroneal artery.

19 D

The artery commences at the lower border of teres major. It initially lies medial to the humerus and then moves anteriorly. Proximally the ulnar nerve is medial to it, and the musculocutaneous and median nerves lie laterally. It lies medial to biceps and its tendon.

20 E

The Hardinge (lateral) approach to the hip splits tensor fascia lata, vastus lateralis and gluteus medius. Piriformis, obturator internus and the gemellae are detached from the greater trochanter in the posterior approach to the hip.

21   D

The ulnar nerve can get trapped in the arcade of Struthers, which is the proximal end of the cubital tunnel. The median and radial nerves pass through the cubital fossa, but not the ulnar. The radial nerve passes through the lateral triangular space and the median nerve through the carpal tunnel. The arcade of Frohse is a site of possible posterior interosseus nerve entrapment.

22   E

The midpoint of the inguinal ligament is half way between the anterior superior iliac spine and the pubic tubercle. The deep inguinal ring and femoral nerve lie at this point. The midinguinal point is half way between the anterior superior iliac spine and the pubic symphysis. The femoral artery lies at this point.

23   D

The boundaries of the inguinal canal are:

- roof – transversus abdominis, internal oblique and the conjoint tendon
- floor – inguinal ligament and lacunar ligament
- anterior – external oblique and internal oblique
- posterior – transversalis fascia and the conjoint tendon

24   B

The saphenous vein passes anterior to the medial malleolus. The structures passing posterior from nearest back are tibia, posterior tendon, flexor digitorum longus tendon, posterior tibial artery, posterior tibial vein, posterior tibial nerve and the flexor hallucis longus tendon.

25   C

The nerves lying in the lateral wall of the cavernous sinus are the oculomotor, trochlear and the ophthalmic and maxillary branches of the trigeminal.

26   E

The muscles attached to the common flexor origin are pronator teres, flexor carpi radialis, palmaris longus, flexor digitorum superficialis and flexor carpi ulnaris. The deep muscles of the forearm do not attach, and they are pronator quadratus, flexor digitorum profundus and flexor pollicis longus.

27   A

Structures passing through the foramen magnum are the medulla, meninges, tectorial membrane, anterior spinal artery, vertebral artery and spinal branches of the accessory nerve.

28   E

The boundaries are:

- superiorly (base) – inguinal ligament
- medially – medial border of adductor longus
- laterally – medial border of sartorius
- floor – adductor longus, pectineus, iliac and psoas
- roof – fascia and skin

29   D

The rectus sheath contains the superior and inferior epigastric arteries and veins, rectus abdominis, pyramidalis and the lower six thoracic nerves.

30   C

The medial longitudinal arch comprises the talus, navicular, calcaneum, cuneiforms and medial three metatarsals. The cuboid is lateral.

31   B

The plane of Louis lies at the lower border of T4, at the level of the second costal cartilage. It divides the mediastinum into superior and inferior. The trachea bifurcates at this level, aorta arches and azygous vein enters the SVC.

32   E

The fourth part of the duodenum lies at the level of L2.

33   A

The sciatic nerve supplies both gemellae, quadratus femoris, semitendinosus, semimembranosus, both heads of biceps femoris, the hamstring half of adductor magnus and obturator internus. Obturator externus is supplied by the obturator nerve.

34   D

The branches of the posterior cord are the upper and lower subscapular nerves, thoracodorsal nerve, axillary nerve and radial nerve. The musculocutaneous nerve is a branch of the lateral cord.

35   D

Apnoeic coma and a known cause of irreversible brain damage are pre-requisites for brainstem death testing. The patient must not be hypothermic, have uncorrected metabolic derangements (except Na in diabetes insipidus), or be under the influence of sedative medications. Tests to be performed are pupil responses, corneal reflexes, a caloric test, gag reflex, apnoea test and pain reflex. However, the pain reflex must be in the facial nerve distribution, as reflexes below the neck may be spinal.

36   D

A Swan–Ganz catheter can be used to directly measure mean arterial pressure, central venous pressure, pulmonary artery wedge pressure, cardiac output (using Fick's principle). Peripheral and systemic vascular resistance and ventricular stroke work are calculated, not directly measured.

37   E

Each gram of haemoglobin binds 1.34 mL of oxygen when fully saturated. The curve is moved to the left by alkaline pH, decreased temperature, decreased $PaCO_2$, decreased 2,3 DPG, fetal haemoglobin and COHb. At a PaO_2 of 40 mmHg the saturation of Hb is 75%; at 26 mmHg the saturation is 50%.

38   E

30% is transported as carbaminohaemoglobin, 10% dissolved in the plasma and 60% transported as sodium bicarbonate. The carbaminohaemoglobin curve never saturates. Carbonic anhydrase catalyses the reaction of CO_2 and plasma.

39   B

CSF is produced by the choroid plexus and reabsorbed by the arachnoid villae. The rate of production is unrelated to the pressure in the ventricles, subarachnoid space, and systemic BP. It passes from the lateral to the third ventricles via the foramen of Munro, and from the third to the fourth ventricles via the aqueduct of Sylvius. It passes into the subarachnoid space via the foramina of Luschka and foramen of Magendie.

40   D

The normal values are tidal volume 500 mL, inspiratory reserve volume 3000 mL, expiratory reserve volume 2000 mL, vital capacity 5600 mL, and total lung capacity 6000 mL.

41   B

1% lignocaine contains 10 mg/mL. The maximum safe dose without adrenaline is 3 mg/kg. The maximum dose is therefore 210 mL, which is contained in 21 mL.

42 C

PTH secretion is decreased by increased serum phosphate, decreased free calcium ions, decreased magnesium and increased $1,25(OH)_2D$. Its secretion is unrelated to serum potassium level.

43 A

The secretions of the adrenal glands by zone are:

- zona glomerulosa – aldosterone
- zona fasiculata – cortisol and testosterone
- zona reticulosa – oestradiol and progesterone
- adrenal medulla – adrenaline, noradrenaline and dopamine

44 E

Hartman's contains 130 mmol of sodium, 111 mmol of chloride, 0 mmol of glucose and 2 mmol of calcium.

45 D

1500 mL of saliva, 2000 mL of gastric secretions, 1000 mL of pancreatic juices, 1500 mL of bile, 3500 mL of small bowel secretions and 500 mL of large bowel secretions are secreted per day.

46   E

Hydrochloric acid is produced by the parietal cells.

47   B

Bile contains conjugated bilirubin with glucouronic acid, which make up the bile pigments. The other constituents are bile salts/acids, inorganic salts (eg sodium chloride and sodium bicarbonate), phospholipids (eg cholesterol and lecithins), and water, which makes up 97% of the bile.

48   D

Factors XII, XI, and IX are all part of the intrinsic pathway. Factor VII is common to both pathways. Factor III is part of the extrinsic pathway. Factor XIII is part of the final common pathway.

49   A

Answers B–E are the main functions of the terminal ileum. Folate reuptake is a function of the jejunum.

50   B

Proaccelerin is a plasma protein. All of the other factors (prothrombin, plasminogen, antithrombin and fibrinogen) are synthesised by the liver, as is factor VIII.

51 B

Renin is secreted by the granular cells of the juxtaglomerular apparatus. In the blood it converts angiotensin to angiotensin I. Angiotensin I is converted to angiotensin II by angiotensin converting enzyme in the lungs. Angiotensin II stimulates aldosterone and antidiuretic hormone. Antidiuretic hormone is produced by the hypothalamus and stored in the posterior pituitary, from which it is released.

52 C

Sodium, glucose, bicarbonate and amino acids are actively reabsorbed in the proximal tubule. Phosphate and calcium are reabsorbed subject to control. Urea and water are passively reabsorbed. Hydrogen ions are secreted dependent on pH.

53 D

The chemoreceptors concerned with blood pressure maintenance are located at the carotid bifurcation and aortic bodies. The stretch receptors are located in the walls of the atria and pulmonary arteries. The chemoreceptors are stimulated by low oxygen levels, high carbon dioxide level and acidic pH. The stretch receptors respond to stretching of the vessel walls.

54 B

The fight or flight response is controlled by the hypothalamus, which controls release of catecholamines from the adrenal medulla. It includes constriction of blood vessels, increased heart rate and increased contraction strength, sweating, decreased GI activity and dilatation of the pupils.

55   C

Sodium, magnesium, calcium and potassium are all cations. Chloride, phosphate, bicarbonate, lactate, sulphate and albumin are all anions.

56   E

The accessory muscles of expiration are the abdominal muscles, which can force the diaphragm upwards by contracting, including rectus abdominis, transverses abdominis, internal and external oblique. Sternocleidomastoid and the scalene muscles are the major accessory muscles of inspiration.

57   D

Vitamin B_{12} is necessary for maturation of red cells; it is stored in the liver and also present in bile. Stores are large and can last 3–6 years. Intrinsic factor secreted by gastric parietal cells is necessary for its uptake.

58   C

Pancreatic polypeptide, somatostatin, glucagons and insulin are endocrine secretions of the pancreas. The exocrine secretions are tripsinogen, chymotrypsinogen, procarboxylase, procarboxypeptidases, phospholipase, amylase and lecithin.

59   E

Compliance is reduced by alveolar oedema, pulmonary hypertension, atelectasis and pulmonary fibrosis. It is increased by emphysema, acute asthma and age.

60   C

The anterior pituitary secretes ACTH, FSH, LH, TSH, GH and prolactin. The posterior pituitary releases ADH.

61   C

1 mmol/kg potassium and chloride, 2 mmol/kg of sodium, 0.1 mmol/kg of calcium, and approximately 35 mL/kg of water are required per day.

62   A

Excess acid intake and excess bicarbonate loss, eg in diarrhoea, are causes of metabolic acidosis with a normal anion gap. The other conditions all cause an increased anion gap.

63   D

CEA is a non-specific marker for a variety of tumours and pathologies, but not for testicular tumours. α-fetoprotein is a marker for NGSCT, but not for pure seminoma.

64   D

There is no proven link between alcohol and bladder cancer; links have been shown to β-naphthamine (in dyes and in cigarette smoke), schistosomiasis, benzidine, aromatic amines and trauma (eg from catheterisation or calculi).

65   D

EBV is known to be carcinogenic for B-cell lymphoma, nasopharyngeal carcinoma and Hodgkin's lymphoma.

66   D

Epstein–Barr virus is linked to B-cell lymphoma, Hodgkin's lymphoma and nasopharyngeal carcinoma. Hepatitis B and C are linked to hepatocellular carcinoma, but no link has been shown to Hepatitis A. HIV is linked to leukaemia, lymphoma and Kaposi sarcoma. HPV is linked to cervical cancer.

67   E

MEN 1 is inherited in an autosomal dominant fashion; the gene is located on chromosome 11; the gene for MEN 2 is on chromosome 10. MEN 2A is known as Sipple's syndrome. Phaeochromocytoma is a common feature of MEN 2B, not MEN 1.

68   E

Gastrinoma is a common feature of MEN 1.

69   E

Meckel's diverticulum is the commonest congenital developmental anomaly, more common in males. It is present in 2% of the population, 2 inches long and 2 feet from the ileocaecal junction. It contains all layers of the intestinal wall. It may contain gastric or pancreatic mucosa. It is a remnant of the omphalomesenteric duct.

70   C

All inhalational anaesthetic agents except nitrous oxide can cause malignant hyperpyrexia, suxamethonium can also cause it. The treatment involves dantrolene. Malignant hyperpyrexia occurs in 1 in 150,000.

71   B

The characteristic features of acute inflammation are dolor (pain), rubor (erythema), tumour (swelling) and calor (heat).

72   D

Tumour markers can be enzymes, hormones, oncofetal antigens and ectopic hormones.

73   E

Answers A–D are characteristics of necrosis. Apoptosis is a physiological process of programmed cell death, which is irreversible once initiated, and energy driven. The cells shrink and are packed into vesicles.

74   A

Blood for transfusion is routinely screened for hepatitis B and C, HIV, CMV and syphilis.

75   C

Psammoma bodies on histology are characteristic of papillary thyroid carcinoma.

76   B

Clostridia are Gram-positive rods, as are *Listeria* and diphtheroids. Examples of Gram-negative rods include *Escherichia coli, Klebsiella, Yersinia, Haemophilus, Pseudomonas, Shigella, Legionella, Proteus* and *Salmonella*.

77   D

Tumours that commonly metastasise to bone are breast, bronchus, thyroid, prostate and kidney.

78   C

Granulomas are found in TB, leprosy, schistosomiasis, syphilis, sarcoidosis and Crohn's disease. The lack of granulomas in ulcerative colitis is one of the differences between the two types of inflammatory bowel disease.

79   D

Dysplasia is a premalignant change. It causes increased cell growth and mitosis. It causes abnormal differentiation with pleomorphism, hyperchromism and high nuclear-to-cytoplasmic ratio.

80   C

Fair skin, albinism, xeroderma pigmentosum and family history are all risk factors for malignant melanoma. Intermittent sun exposure is a risk factor, with stronger links between continuous exposure and basal cell and squamous cell carcinoma.

81   D

Pott's peculiar tumour is a trichilemmal cyst; a harmatoma is an overgrowth of one or more cell types that are normally present. A turban tumour is a type of cylindroma and seborrhoeic keratoses are a benign overgrowth of the basal layer of the epidermis.

82   B

Vitamin A is required for epithelial cell proliferation. Vitamin B_6 is required for collagen cross-links. Zinc is required for RNA and DNA synthesis. Copper is required for cross-linking of collagen.

83   D

Platelets appear immediately in a wound, followed by neutrophils within a day. Macrophages appear within 2 days, then fibroblasts and myofibroblasts in 2–4 days, then endothelial cells in 3–5 days.

84   E

Hypertrophy is an increase in cell size, and hyperplasia is an increase in cell number. Metaplasia is the conversion of one tissue type to another. Teratoma is a growth of cells originating from more than one germ cell line. Hamartoma is an overgrowth of cell normally found in that tissue.

85   A

Squamous carcinoma is the most common type, followed by small cell, adenocarcinoma large cell and adenosquamous.

86   E

Pleomorphic adenoma is the commonest salivary gland tumour. It is benign, although a small number undergo malignant transformation. It is commonest in the parotid gland, but can occur in any salivary gland. It is commoner in males most often presenting in the fourth and fifth decades. 10% of Warthin's tumours are bilateral.

87   A

Reed–Sternberg cells are characteristic of Hodgkin's lymphoma.

88   C

Known risk factors for hepatocellular carcinoma include hepatitis B and C aflatoxin, anabolic steroids, alcohol cirrhosis and primary liver disease.

89   C

Local factors delaying wound healing include infection, haematoma, foreign bodies, decreased blood supply and poor surgical technique. Malnutrition does affect wound healing, but is a systemic factor.

90   E

Infantile hypertrophic pyloric stenosis is present in 31,000 live births. It is more common in first born males and usually presents between 3 and 6 weeks.

PRACTICE PAPER 5: QUESTIONS

PRACTICE PAPER 5: QUESTIONS

1   **Which of the following micro-organisms is correctly paired with its description?**

○   A   *Clostridium difficile* – Gram-negative cocci – aerobic

○   B   *Streptococcus faecalis* – Gram-positive cocci – aerobic

○   C   *Bacillus* species – Gram-negative bacilli – aerobic

○   D   *Actinomyces israelii* – Gram-positive bacilli – aerobic

○   E   *Escherichia coli* – Gram-negative bacilli – anaerobic

2   **A 49-year-old woman presents to A+E with severe left-sided abdominal pain, which becomes generalised with fever. CT scan confirms perforated diverticulum, and she is prepared for theatre. Which of the following descriptions best describes the type of wound created by the required operation?**

○   A   clean wound

○   B   clean-contaminated wound

○   C   contaminated wound

○   D   dirty wound

○   E   none of the above

3 Which of the following hereditary immune disorders is NOT correctly paired with the affected component of the immune system?

- ⃝ A Chronic Granulomatous Disease (CGD) – macrophages
- ⃝ B DiGeorge syndrome – T-cells
- ⃝ C Leucocyte Adhesion Deficiency (LAD) – neutrophils
- ⃝ D hereditary angioedema – complement pathway
- ⃝ E X-linked hypogammaglobulinaemia – B-cells

4 An example of a depolarising muscle relaxant used in anaesthesia is

- ⃝ A vecuronium
- ⃝ B gallamine
- ⃝ C propofol
- ⃝ D suxamethonium
- ⃝ E neostigmine

5 The correct 'shelf-life' of platelet concentrates is

- ⃝ A 4°C, maximum 35 days
- ⃝ B room temperature, maximum 5 days
- ⃝ C –30°C, maximum 12 months
- ⃝ D –65°C, maximum 3 years
- ⃝ E room temperature, maximum 24 hours

6   Autologous blood transfusion is contraindicated in all of the following conditions EXCEPT

- ○ A   hepatitis B
- ○ B   severe hypertension
- ○ C   steroid use
- ○ D   unstable angina
- ○ E   aortic stenosis

7   A patient has blood sent away for clotting studies and the results show a raised prothrombin time, but APTT, thrombin time and platelet count are normal. What is the most likely reason?

- ○ A   heparin treatment
- ○ B   liver disease
- ○ C   disseminated intravascular coagulation
- ○ D   warfarin treatment
- ○ E   vitamin K treatment

8   A patient arrives in A+E with the following arterial blood gases results: PaO_2 8.0; $PaCO_2$ 2.0; pH 7.54; bicarbonate 18. The most likely cause is

- ○ A   excessive vomiting
- ○ B   PE
- ○ C   diabetic ketoacidosis
- ○ D   CVA
- ○ E   chest wall trauma

9 The correct composition of 'Hartman's solution' is as follows

		Na	Cl	Dextrose	K	PO$_4$	Ca	HCO$_3$
○	A	154	154	–	20	–	2	18
○	B	131	111	–	5	–	2	29
○	C	129	109	–	4	1.5	–	29
○	D	30	30	222	2	–	2	–
○	E	147	156	–	4	–	2.2	–

all in mmol/L

10 Which of the following medications is NOT known to cause renal failure?

○ A diclofenac

○ B ciprofloxacin

○ C simvastatin

○ D frusemide

○ E mannitol

11 Which of the following blood results is most likely to indicate recent infection with hepatitis B?

		HBsAg	HBeAg	Anti HBsAg	Anti-HBcAg
○	A	–	–	+	+
○	B	–	+	–	+
○	C	+	–	+	–
○	D	+	+	–	+
○	E	+	+	+	+

12 A 24-year-old motorcyclist has a collision with a car and is thrown 2 metres, landing on his head. When assessed at the scene he is mumbling incoherently, moving in response to command and opening his eyes only in response to painful stimuli. His GCS score is

○ A 9
○ B 10
○ C 6
○ D 12
○ E 8

13   A 70 kg man (blood volume 5 litres) is involved in a road traffic
accident and fractures his femur. On arrival at hospital he is
confused and tachycardic at 130 bpm. Other measurements are
BP 80/40, respiratory rate 34, urine output 5 mL/hour. Most
probable amount of blood loss is

○   A   750 mL

○   B   1200 mL

○   C   2500 mL

○   D   500 mL

○   E   1750 mL

14   Select the one suture type that is not paired with its appropriate
description.

○   A   polypropylene (prolene) – non-absorbable, synthetic,
monofilament

○   B   silk – non-absorbable, natural, multifilament

○   C   polyester – absorbable, synthetic, multifilament

○   D   polyglecaprine (PDS) – absorbable, synthetic, monofilament

○   E   polyglactin (vicryl) – absorbable, synthetic, multifilament

15   A patient requires removal of sebaceous cyst from his scalp under
local anaesthesia. Which preparation is most appropriate?

○   A   lignocaine and adrenaline 5 mg/kg

○   B   prilocaine 2 mg/kg

○   C   bupivicaine 6 mg/kg

○   D   lignocaine 5 mg/kg

○   E   bupivicaine and adrenaline 2 mg/kg

16 Which one of the following statements are correct regarding the movements of breathing?

○ A   expiration is primarily due to active contraction of the internal intercostals

○ B   movement of ribs 2–7 is a 'pump handle' type action, which increases the anterior–posterior diameter of the thorax

○ C   movement of ribs 8–12 increases the vertical diameter of the thorax

○ D   the first rib moves laterally during inspiration

○ E   contraction of the diaphragm aids expiration

17 Which one of the following statements about the anatomy of the heart is false?

○ A   the anterior cardiac veins drain into the right atrium

○ B   the fossa ovalis may remain patent in 10% of normal subjects

○ C   the sinus venosus forms part of the ventricular walls

○ D   the sino-atrial node lies in the upper end of the crista terminalis

○ E   the aorta is derived from the truncus arteriosus

18 Which one of the following statements about the great vessels is true?

○ A the left brachiocephalic artery divides to form the left common carotid artery and left subclavian artery

○ B the right subclavian vein and right internal jugular vein join to form the right brachiocephalic trunk

○ C the left internal jugular vein drains directly into the superior vena cava

○ D the right common carotid artery arises directly from the aortic arch

○ E the IVC joins the SVC before draining into the right atrium

19 Which one of the following statements about the abdominal aorta and its branches is true?

○ A the inferior mesenteric artery lies at the level of L2

○ B the gonadal arteries arise beneath the renal arteries

○ C the common iliac artery divides into three branches

○ D the median sacral artery arises at L3

○ E there are five lumbar arteries

20 Which of the following statements about the relations of the kidney and adrenal glands is false?

○ A the duodenum overlies the hilum of the right kidney

○ B the adrenals lie within the renal fascia

○ C the small intestine overlies the inferior pole of both kidneys

○ D the hila of both kidneys lies at the approximate level of L3

○ E there are five segmental branches from each renal artery

21 **Which statement is true regarding the axilla?**

○ A pectoralis major forms the posterior wall

○ B latissimus dorsi forms the lateral wall

○ C the apex is bounded by the first rib, clavicle and scapula

○ D serratus anterior contributes to forming the posterior wall

○ E the floor of the axilla is formed by the clavipectoral fascia

22 **Which statement is true regarding the compartments of the lower leg?**

○ A the nerve within the anterior compartment is the deep peroneal nerve

○ B flexor hallucis longus lies within the anterior compartment

○ C the posterior compartment is divided into deep and superficial parts by the interosseous membrane

○ D soleus is within the deep posterior compartment

○ E the tibial nerve runs through the lateral compartment

23 **A man is involved in a road traffic accident and injures his left leg. Following the injury he finds himself unable to extend the left knee and notices loss of sensation along the medial side of the lower leg up to the big toe. The likely nerve injured is**

○ A sciatic nerve

○ B tibial nerve

○ C femoral nerve

○ D common peroneal nerve

○ E superficial peroneal nerve

24   A man is stabbed in the arm during a fight. On examination he finds himself unable to extend his wrist, although his elbow movement is intact. The injury is most likely to involve

○   A   the radial nerve in the axilla

○   B   the median nerve as it passes between heads of pronator teres

○   C   the ulnar nerve as it passes behind the median epicondyle

○   D   the radial nerve in the spiral groove

○   E   the median nerve as it arises from the lateral and medial cords of the brachial plexus

25   Which of the following statements about the femoral canal is false?

○   A   it contains a lymph node called Cloquet's node

○   B   the femoral nerve lies laterally within the canal

○   C   the femoral sheath is derived from extraperitoneal, intra-abdominal fascia

○   D   it serves as a pathway for lower limb lymphatics

○   E   it is approximately 0.5 cm wide

26   Which statement is true regarding the parotid gland?

○   A   tumours of the gland can result in sensory loss of the affected side of the face

○   B   the parotid duct pierces buccinator opposite the 2nd lower molar tooth

○   C   the retromandibular vein passes through the gland

○   D   the external carotid artery lies deep to the gland

○   E   the gland overlies the anterior belly of the digastric muscle

27   Which of the following statements about the larynx is true?

○   A   the top of the thyroid cartilage lies at the level of C3

○   B   the cricoid cartilage is a derivative of the VIth arch

○   C   all the intrinsic muscles except cricothyroid are supplied by the superior laryngeal nerve

○   D   the hyoid bone lies at the level of C2

○   E   the posterior cricoarytenoids close the vocal cords together

28   Which statement is true regarding the surface anatomy of the abdomen?

○   A   the gallbladder lies at the level of the 10th costal cartilage in the midclavicular line

○   B   the neck of the pancreas lies at L2

○   C   the superior pole of the kidney lies at the level of the 9th rib posteriorly

○   D   the transpyloric plane of Addison lies half way between the suprasternal notch and the iliac crests

○   E   the spleen lies over the 9th, 10th and 11th ribs posteriorly

29   Which one of the following statements about the diaphragm is false?

○   A   it attaches to the xiphoid

○   B   the left crus arises from L1–2

○   C   the left phrenic nerve pierces the diaphragm together with the IVC at the level of T8

○   D   the aorta pierces the diaphragm at T12

○   E   it arises from the lower six costal cartilages laterally

30 **Which statement is true regarding the bladder?**

○ A sympathetic fibres cause relaxation of the detrusor muscle and contraction of the internal sphincter

○ B in the male, the external sphincter lies above the prostate

○ C it receives its blood supply from branches of the external iliac arteries

○ D it is entirely covered by peritoneum

○ E the trigone is situated at the apex of the bladder

31 **Which of the following features is NOT associated with a full thickness burn?**

○ A black/white colour

○ B reduced blanching

○ C no sensation

○ D usually requiring treatment with skin graft

○ E minimal healing

32 **A woman is brought to A+E after being rescued from a house fire. She has burns affecting her left arm and anterior surfaces of both legs. Using Wallace's Rule of Nines the percentage of area burnt is**

○ A 45%

○ B 18%

○ C 36%

○ D 27%

○ E 54%

33   Damage to peripheral nerves results in specific areas of sensory loss. Which of the following nerve–sensory area pairings is incorrect?

◯   A   radial nerve – dorsal web space between thumb and index finger

◯   B   musculocutaneous nerve – lateral area of forearm

◯   C   median nerve – palmar aspect of index finger

◯   D   obturator nerve – lateral aspect of thigh

◯   E   deep peroneal nerve – dorsal aspect of 1st web space

34   Which of the following is NOT a complication of mechanical ventilation?

◯   A   pneumothorax

◯   B   gastric dilatation

◯   C   acute respiratory distress syndrome (ARDS)

◯   D   atrophy of respiratory muscles

◯   E   reduced venous return

35   Which of the following is NOT a feature of acute respiratory distress syndrome (ARDS)?

◯   A   severe hypoxaemia (PaO_2/FiO_2 <27)

◯   B   pulmonary infiltrates on chest X-ray

◯   C   a known cause (eg pancreatitis)

◯   D   cardiac pulmonary oedema

◯   E   pulmonary artery wedge pressure (PAWP) <18mmHg

36 A man presents to A+E with a very low urine output. Analysis of urine and serum samples gives the following results: urinary sodium 15 mmol/L; urine osmolarity 520; urine:serum osmolarity ratio 1.5. Most likely cause is

- A   bilateral PUJ obstruction
- B   retention secondary to enlarged prostate
- C   excessive diarrhoea and vomiting
- D   interstitial nephritis
- E   glomerulonephritis

37 Which of the following is NOT a test used to determine brainstem death?

- A   corneal reflex
- B   gag reflex
- C   caloric test
- D   pain reflex
- E   flexor response

38 Which of the following is NOT used in the definition of systemic inflammatory response syndrome (SIRS)?

- A   temperature >39°C
- B   tachycardia >90 bpm
- C   temperature <36°C
- D   bradycardia <45 bpm
- E $PaCO_2$ <4.3 kPa

39 A tumour marker used in surveillance after orchidectomy for non-seminomatous germ cell tumours of the testes is

○ A   prostate-specific antigen (PSA)

○ B   alpha-fetoprotein

○ C   carcinoma CA–125

○ D   carcinoembryonic antigen (CEA)

○ E   CA 19–9

40 Which of the following is NOT a feature of multiple endocrine neoplasia type II?

○ A   medullary thyroid cancer

○ B   phaeochromocytoma

○ C   pituitary adenoma

○ D   parathyroid tumours

○ E   multiple mucosal neuromas

41 Which of the following is an appropriate clearance margin for removal of a squamous cell carcinoma of the skin?

○ A   1–2 cm

○ B   5 cm

○ C   0.5 cm

○ D   3–4 cm

○ E   2 mm

42   **A woman presents with a green discharge from her nipple. Most likely diagnosis is**

○   A   carcinoma of the breast

○   B   lactating breast

○   C   duct ectasia

○   D   breast abscess

○   E   duct papilloma

43   **Which of the following is NOT a risk factor for breast cancer?**

○   A   affected sister

○   B   Li–Fraumeni syndrome

○   C   multiparity

○   D   obesity

○   E   early menarche

44   **A woman with suspected breast cancer has fine needle aspiration of a breast lump. The report comes back as 'C3'. What does this mean?**

○   A   equivocal

○   B   suspicious for cancer

○   C   inadequate sample

○   D   definitely malignant

○   E   benign

45   Which of the following statements about coronary circulation is false?

○   A   most of the perfusion of the left ventricle occurs during diastole

○   B   direction of blood flow to the myocardium is from the outer surface of the heart inwards

○   C   changes in blood flow in the coronary arteries occurs by auto-regulation

○   D   the interventricular septum is supplied by the left coronary artery only

○   E   the right coronary artery arises from the right aortic sinus

46   A man is found to have a PSA of 14 on routine testing. He is entirely asymptomatic. Investigation with transrectal biopsy confirms prostate cancer. MRI scan shows a nodule on the left lobe, which extends into the seminal vesicles. The stage of prostate cancer based on this information is

○   A   T4

○   B   T3a

○   C   T2a

○   D   T3b

○   E   T2b

47 Which of the following agents used in the treatment of urological conditions is NOT paired with its correct description?

◯ A   mitomycin C – intravesical chemotherapy agent

◯ B   finasteride – luteinising hormone-releasing hormone (LH-RH) agonist

◯ C   oxybutinin – anticholinergic agent

◯ D   tamsulosin – α-adrenergic blocker

◯ E   flutamide – anti-androgen agent

48 A man is found to have a hydrocele, which at operation is found to extend from the testes to the deep inguinal ring, but not connect with the peritoneal cavity. Which of the following best describes this hydrocele?

◯ A   vaginal hydrocele

◯ B   congenital hydrocele

◯ C   infantile hydrocele

◯ D   hydrocele of cord

◯ E   malignant hydrocele

49 A 15-year-old boy presents with sudden onset right testicular pain
associated with nausea and vomiting. On examination, the right
testis is found to be drawn up into the groin with a horizontal lie
and is very tender. What is the most appropriate form of
management?

○ A broad spectrum antibiotics

○ B exploration of testis via inguinal incision

○ C bed rest and scrotal support

○ D 'watch and wait' policy

○ E exploration of testis via transverse incision over testis

50 All of the following are complications of transurethral resection of
prostate (TURP), EXCEPT

○ A urethral stricture

○ B retrograde ejaculation

○ C hypernatraemia

○ D incontinence

○ E increased risk of myocardial infarction

51 **Which statement is TRUE regarding the rotator cuff?**

○ A teres minor is attached to the lesser tuberosity

○ B the muscles attach at the level of the surgical neck of the humerus

○ C the tendon of infraspinatus is fused with the capsule of the shoulder joint

○ D subscapularis runs through a tunnel formed by the acromion and the coraco-acromial ligament

○ E it supports the shoulder joint but is deficient inferiorly

52 **Which of the following statements about hernias is TRUE?**

○ A paraumbilical hernias are usually congenital

○ B lumbar hernias usually present as an emergency with strangulation

○ C a hernia containing a strangulated Meckel's diverticulum is a Littre's hernia

○ D femoral hernias appear below and medial to the pubic tubercle

○ E Spigelian hernias generally occur through the epiploic foramen of Winslow

53 **All of the following statements about radiotherapy are true EXCEPT:**

○ A   it can be administered via X-rays

○ B   the nature of the surrounding tissue influences how much radiotherapy is administered

○ C   multiple fractions are required for palliation of bone pain

○ D   seminomas are very sensitive to radiotherapy

○ E   ulceration is a recognised complication

54 **The following statements regarding lung function tests are true EXCEPT:**

○ A   the functional residual capacity is made up of the residual volume and expiratory reserve volume

○ B   in an average 20-year-old male, tidal volume is approximately 0.5 litres

○ C   the residual volume is the amount of air remaining in the lungs after maximum expiration

○ D   total lung capacity is the sum of residual volume and tidal volume

○ E   vital capacity can be measured by spirometry

55   Which of the following statements about arterial ulcers is NOT true?

○   A   they are often found at tips of toes

○   B   the foot may show venous guttering

○   C   they are associated with lipodermatosclerosis

○   D   they are painful

○   E   they have 'punched out' appearance

56   Risks associated with carotid endarterectomy include all of the following EXCEPT

○   A   stroke

○   B   myocardial infarction (MI)

○   C   wound infection

○   D   damage to the accessory nerve

○   E   damage to the glossopharyngeal nerve

57   A 60-year-old man presents with a history of claudication pain in his left leg after walking 20 metres which is impacting significantly on his lifestyle. He is investigated by arteriography, which shows an 2 cm stenosis in the proximal superficial femoral artery. Most appropriate management is

○   A   below knee amputation

○   B   correction of risk factors only

○   C   percutaneous balloon angioplasty

○   D   femoropopliteal bypass

○   E   femorodistal bypass

58 A man presents with left buttock, thigh and calf claudication pain. Where is the most likely site of arterial disease?

- ○ A left superficial femoral artery
- ○ B left common iliac artery
- ○ C left external iliac artery
- ○ D left internal iliac artery
- ○ E lower aorta

59 Which of the following statements about abdominal aortic aneurysms is TRUE?

- ○ A they can can be stented if above the renal arteries
- ○ B they are operated on when <5.5 cm in diameter
- ○ C they may cause emboli
- ○ D they are not identified on ultrasound scan
- ○ E they are more common in females

60 All of the statements about lymphoedema are correct EXCEPT

- ○ A it may be a primary problem
- ○ B malignant infiltration of lymphatics is a common cause of secondary lymphoedema
- ○ C it may occur secondary to radiotherapy
- ○ D ulceration in primary lymphoedema is common
- ○ E operative treatment is rarely used

61 A 4-year-old girl falls from her bike landing on her left leg, which becomes tender and swollen. X-ray shows a fracture of the proximal tibia, which goes through a radiolucent area with a well-defined sclerotic edge. Most likely diagnosis is

- ○ A osteosarcoma
- ○ B chondrosarcoma
- ○ C bone cyst
- ○ D bone metastasis
- ○ E Ewing's sarcoma

62 A 40-year-old diabetic man presents with pain in the upper lumbar spine. X-ray at the time showed soft tissue swelling only and he was discharged home with anti-inflammatories. He returns 10 days later as his symptoms are no better and he has been suffering from a constant fever. X-ray at this time shows sclerotic changes and periosteal reaction. His symptoms are most likely due to infection with:

- ○ A *Salmonella*
- ○ B *Haemophilus influenzae*
- ○ C *Gonococcus*
- ○ D tuberculosis
- ○ E *Staphylococcus aureus*

63   The following are all features of carpal tunnel syndrome EXCEPT

○   A   pain often worse at night

○   B   positive Tinel's test

○   C   positive Phalen's test

○   D   wasting of the hypothenar muscles

○   E   paraesthesia over thumb and lateral two fingers

64   All of the following may be radiological features of osteoarthritis EXCEPT

○   A   bone cysts

○   B   subchondral sclerosis

○   C   osteophytes

○   D   increased joint space

○   E   joint effusion

65   Which of the following statements about the popliteal fossa is TRUE?

○   A   the lateral edge is bounded by semimembranosus and gastrocnemius

○   B   the deep fascia forms the roof and is pierced by the long saphenous vein

○   C   the popliteal artery is the deepest structure within the fossa

○   D   the common peroneal nerve lies medially within the fossa

○   E   soleus forms the medial lower edge

66 Which of the following statements about the brachial plexus is FALSE?

- A   the thoracodorsal nerve arises from the posterior cord
- B   the medial and lateral cords join to form the median nerve
- C   the trunks of the plexus are found in the posterior triangle of the neck
- D   the long thoracic nerve originate from trunks C5, C6 and C7
- E   the nerve that supplies subscapularis is a branch from the posterior cord

67 A 26-year-old woman is involved in a road traffic accident. On arrival in A+E she has a painful deformed looking left leg which is shortened and internally rotated. She is unable to dorsiflex or plantar flex her foot and there is sensory loss below the knee apart from the medial leg and foot and upper, back of the calf. The nerve most likely to have been affected is

- A   obturator nerve
- B   sciatic nerve
- C   femoral nerve
- D   tibial nerve
- E   common peroneal nerve

68 A 35-year-old tennis player finds herself unable to play because of a painful left shoulder. Pain is worse on lifting the arm, particularly when elevated between 60–120 degrees. On examination there is tenderness just lateral to the acromium process. The diagnosis is

- ○ A   supraspinatus rupture
- ○ B   frozen shoulder
- ○ C   acromioclavicular joint dislocation
- ○ D   supraspinatus tendonitis
- ○ E   biceps tendon rupture

69 All of the following statements about a fractured neck of femur are true EXCEPT

- ○ A   the affected leg is shortened and externally rotated
- ○ B   associated mortality is in the region of >30% at 6 months
- ○ C   intertrochanteric fractures are usually fixed using a dynamic hip screw
- ○ D   intracapsular fractures may result in avascular necrosis of the femoral head
- ○ E   femoral nerve injury is common

70 A 67-year-old man presents extremely unwell with left-sided abdominal pain, fever and shock. At emergency laparotomy he is found to have a large tumour of the sigmoid colon, which has perforated causing faecal contamination. What is the most appropriate operation?

○ A   left hemicolectomy and primary anastomosis

○ B   sigmoid colectomy

○ C   Hartman's procedure

○ D   anterior resection

○ E   abdominoperineal resection

71 Which of the following is NOT a possible long-term complication of gastrectomy?

○ A   bolus obstruction

○ B   dumping

○ C   weight gain

○ D   vitamin B_{12} deficiency

○ E   low serum calcium

72 Which of the following is true about the differences between jejunum and ileum?

○ A   the ileum has a thicker wall than the jejunum

○ B   the jejunum has fewer arterial arcades

○ C   the ileum has a wider lumen

○ D   the jejunum has fewer villi on its inner surface

○ E   the ileum has more valvulae coniventes

73   Which of the following is NOT a feature of ulcerative colitis?

○   A   crypt abscesses

○   B   granulomas

○   C   perianal infection

○   D   pseudopolyps

○   E   backwash ileitis

74   A 69-year-old man presents with mechanical bowel obstruction confirmed by barium enema. Which of the following is NOT a possible cause?

○   A   diverticular disease

○   B   angiodysplasia

○   C   Crohn's disease

○   D   gallstones

○   E   carcinoma of the colon

75   Which of the following is NOT a cause of constipation?

○   A   volvulus

○   B   fissure in ano

○   C   digoxin

○   D   aspirin

○   E   cerebral vascular accident (CVA)

76 A patient with a diagnosis of inflammatory bowel disease may have the following extraintestinal manifestations EXCEPT

○ A episcleritis

○ B sclerosing cholangitis

○ C ankylosing spondylitis

○ D erythema nodosum

○ E sarcoidosis

77 Which of the following is NOT part of the Glasgow Scale to assess the severity of pancreatitis on initial assessment?

○ A white cell count >15 (10^9/L

○ B PaO_2 <60 mmHg

○ C age >55 years

○ D glucose <10 mmol/L

○ E lactate dehydrogenase (LDH) >600 units/L

78 Which of the following is NOT a cause of splenomegaly?

○ A syphilis

○ B polycythaemia

○ C congestive cardiac failure

○ D familial adenomatous polyposis

○ E amyloidosis

79 A 46-year-old woman presents with a small mass to the left of the hyoid bone and anterior to the sternocleidomastoid muscle. It is smooth and compressible and mobile in the horizontal but not vertical plane. There is also a bruit. Probable diagnosis is

○ A   sternomastoid tumour

○ B   dermoid cyst

○ C   carotid body tumour

○ D   laryngocoele

○ E   cystic hygroma

80 Which of the following is NOT a possible complication of thyroidectomy?

○ A   laryngeal oedema

○ B   hypercalcaemia

○ C   hypothyroidism

○ D   haematoma

○ E   superior laryngeal nerve palsy

81 Which of the following systemic conditions is NOT associated with pruritus ani?

○ A   cell-mediated lympholysis (CML)

○ B   systemic lupus erythematosus (SLE)

○ C   obstructive jaundice

○ D   diabetes

○ E   lymphoma

82 Which of the following statements about salivary gland tumours is FALSE?

○ A 80% of parotid gland tumours are benign

○ B 15% of salivary gland neoplasms are submandibular

○ C excision of the submandibular gland may result in Frey's syndrome

○ D malignant parotid tumours may cause facial nerve palsy

○ E adenolymphoma of the parotid (Warthin's tumour) is benign

83 A 73-year-old woman presents with a lump in her neck. Biopsy and imaging indicates that this is an early anaplastic thyroid tumour. What is the most appropriate management?

○ A radiotherapy

○ B chemotherapy

○ C resection and radiotherapy

○ D total thyroidectomy only

○ E radiotherapy and chemotherapy

84 The following endocrine conditions are paired with the correct hormone abnormality EXCEPT

○ A Cushing's syndrome – excess glucocorticoid

○ B phaeochromocytoma – excess catecholamines

○ C Conn's disease – excess adrenocorticotropic hormone (ACTH)

○ D Addison's disease – reduced cortisol secretion

○ E congenital adrenal hyperplasia – 2,1 hydroxylase deficiency

85   A 55-year-old woman treated for 6 months with carbimazole for thyrotoxicosis is no longer getting any control of her symptoms. What is the most appropriate form of management?

○   A   subtotal thyroidectomy

○   B   total thyroidectomy

○   C   radio-iodide treatment

○   D   propylthiouracil

○   E   propranolol

86   The following statements about the anatomy of the orbit are false EXCEPT

○   A   all the muscles that move the eye originate from a fibrous ring except lateral rectus

○   B   the ethmoid bone forms the lateral wall

○   C   the wings of the sphenoid form the posterior wall

○   D   the lateral rectus is supplied by cranial nerve III

○   E   the frontal bone forms the medial wall

87   A 42-year-old opera singer presents with a laryngeal carcinoma of the vocal cord. Staging investigations show this to be limited to the vocal cord with no evidence of spread. What is the most appropriate form of management?

○   A   chemotherapy alone

○   B   radiotherapy alone

○   C   radiotherapy and chemotherapy

○   D   partial laryngectomy

○   E   endoscopic resection

88   The following statements about anatomy of the thyroid gland are all true EXCEPT

○   A   the superior thyroid artery supplies the upper pole

○   B   the inferior thyroid artery is a branch of the external carotid artery

○   C   the isthmus of the gland overlies the 2nd and 3rd tracheal cartilages

○   D   the inferior thyroid vein drains into the brachiocephalic veins

○   E   there may be a pyramidal lobe

89   Following splenectomy, which of the following organisms may cause overwhelming sepsis?

○   A   *Pseudomonas* species

○   B   fungal infections

○   C   *Neisseria meningitidis*

○   D   *Salmonella*

○   E   *Staphylococcus aureus*

90   A 16-year-old boy is hit over the head with a bat while playing cricket. He loses consciousness for 10 minutes but then recovers and wants to carry on playing. His parents take him to the hospital, which is an hour's drive away. On arrival he is drowsy with a GCS of 12. Most likely diagnosis is

○   A   basal skull fracture

○   B   subdural haemorrhage

○   C   extradural haematoma

○   D   subarachnoid haemorrhage

○   E   diffuse axonal injury

PRACTICE PAPER 5: ANSWERS AND TEACHING NOTES

PRACTICE PAPER 5: ANSWERS AND TEACHING NOTES

1   B

Bacteria can be classified in terms of their shape (eg rods or cocci) and the colour they become on Gram staining (pink = positive, blue = negative). They can also be classified according to whether they are aerobes or anaerobes. In the example, all are incorrectly paired apart from B. The correct descriptions are: *C. difficile* – Gram-positive rod anaerobic; *Bacillus* species – Gram-positive rod aerobic; *Actinomyces israelii* – Gram-positive anaerobic; *E. coli* – Gram-positive bacillus (facultative anaerobe).

2   D

Wounds can be classified according to the risk of wound contamination. Clean operations are those that are carried out through sterile uninfected skin, where the GI, GU and respiratory tract are not breached; clean-contaminated is when there is breaching of a hollow viscus other than the colon; contaminated is when contamination of the wound has occurred, eg from a bite or opening of the colon; finally, dirty operations are those in which the operation is carried out in the presence of pus or a perforated viscus. The example used in the question – a perforated diverticulum – would most likely require a Hartman's operation and would be classified as dirty.

3   A

CGD is an inherited deficiency in one subunit of NADPH oxidase used by phagocytes, thus causing patients to develop severe infections from bacteria such as *Staphylococcus aureus* and *Klebsiella*. DiGeorge syndrome is due to failure of development of the 3rd and 4th pharyngeal pouches and therefore results in development of a hypoplastic thymus causing T-cell deficiency. LAD is a result of defects in the beta chain of beta-2 integrins, which are important for leucocyte movement. This results in recurrent infections from extracellular bacteria owing to defective opsonisation, adhesion mobility and chemotaxis. Hereditary angioedema is due to a defect in the C1 inhibitor, and X-linked hypogammaglobulinaemia is due to a block in the maturation of the B cell, which results in recurrent pyogenic infections.

4   D

Suxamethonium is an example of a depolarising muscle relaxant. It has a structure similar to acetylcholine, and acts in a similar way at the neuromuscular junction. Non-depolarising agents include gallamine and vecuronium, which have a slower onset but longer duration of action. Neostigmine is an agent used to reverse non-depolarising neuromuscular blockade. Propofol is an induction agent.

5   B

Platelet transfusions are used for various reasons, for example to correct thrombocytopenia prior to an operation. They should be ABO compatible. They have a shelf-life of 5 days at room temperature. In contrast, red blood cell concentrates have a shelf life of 35 days at 4°C, fresh frozen plasma (FFP) can be stored for a maximum of 12 months at −30°C and granulocytes can be kept for 24 hours at room temperature.

6   C

Autologous blood transfusion is the use of a patient's own blood for transfusion. It may be collected in advance of surgery, immediately prior to surgery or from blood lost intraoperatively. Contraindications for this type of transfusion include active infection, severe hypertension, unstable angina and aortic stenosis.

7   D

Prothrombin time (PT) assesses the extrinsic factor VII as well as the common pathway factors. Activated partial thromboplastin time (APTT) assesses both intrinsic and common pathway factors, and thrombin time (TT) detects a deficiency of fibrinogen or inhibition of thrombin. In the question, the PT is elevated alone. This is most likely to be due to warfarin administration, which blocks the synthesis of vitamin K-dependent factors (II, VII, IX). Heparin treatment causes a raised APTT and TT by binding and activating antithrombin III, therefore reducing fibrin formation. Liver disease results in a reduction in the synthesis of all the coagulation factors except VIII and also impairs absorption of vitamin K. There is therefore raised APTT and PT and also reduced platelets. Disseminated intravascular coagulation (DIC) is a pathological response to many disorders, for example malignancy and infections. It involves haemolysis of red blood cells, fibrinolysis and consumption of haemostatic factors. It therefore results in elevated PT, APTT, TT and reduced levels of platelets.

8   B

The example shows a patient with low PaO_2, low $PaCO_2$, high pH and low bicarbonate. When $PaCO_2$ is low, it shifts the following equilibrium to the left

$$CO_2 + H_2O <> H_2CO_3 <> H^+ + HCO_3^-$$

therefore reducing the concentration of H^+ and causing a respiratory alkalosis. From the given examples, PE is the most likely cause as this results in hyperventilation, which 'blows off' and therefore reduces blood levels of CO_2 but at the same time fails to achieve satisfactory oxygenation.

9   B

Hartman's solution is a crystalloid solution composed of Na 131 mmol/L; K 5 mmol/L; HCO_3 29 mmol/L; Cl 111 mmol/L and Ca 2 mmol/L, which is isotonic with body fluid. As its composition is near physiological, it is commonly used intraoperatively to replace fluid losses.

10   C

Drugs can cause renal failure through a variety of mechanisms. Those that have a direct tubular effect include aminoglycosides, mannitol, NSAIDs, ACE inhibitors and cyclosporine. Sulphonamides and acyclovir can cause tubular obstruction, and beta lactam antibiotics, vancomycin, ciprofloxacin and frusemide can cause acute interstitial nephritis. Acute glomerulonephritis is a recognised complication of penacillamine use. Simvastatin is not known to cause renal impairment.

11   D

Hepatitis B is a hepadnavirus, which is a DNA virus. In the acute phase of infection, the virus releases its surface antigen (HBsAg) into the blood. This is also found to be present in persistent/chronic infections. The core antigen (HBcAg) causes production of HBc antibodies, which are the first antibodies to occur in the course of the infection. It is present in the blood in the brief period when HBsAg disappears and before Hbs antibodies appear, and thus it is an important diagnostic indicator of early infection. HBsAb confers immunity to the HBV virus. The 'e' antigen (HBeAg) is also found in the core of the virus and its presence in the blood indicates active viral production and infection. The antibody against HBeAG (HBeAb) is found at a much later stage of infection.

12   B

The Glasgow coma scale is a system used to record and monitor a patient's level of consciousness. There are a total of 15 points based on three categories:

- best motor response (6 = obeys commands; 5 = localises to pain; 4 = withdraws from pain; 3 = abnormal flexion; 2 = abnormal extension; 1 = none)
- best verbal response (5 = orientated; 4 = confused; 3 = inappropriate speech; 2 = incomprehensible sounds; 1 = none)
- best eye opening response (4 = open spontaneously; 3 = opens to speech; 2 = opens to painful stimulus ; 1 = none).

A GCS of 8 is an important score as it is at this point that you consider a patient for intubation as they are unlikely to be able to protect their own airway.

13 E

Loss of blood volume is associated with physiological responses, mainly mediated by the sympathetic nervous system, which aim to maintain blood pressure and hence blood supply to vital organs. Haemorrhagic shock can be divided into four classes depending on the amount of blood lost. Each class is associated with particular parameters that help in the estimation of blood loss.

- Class 1 is loss of 0–15% of circulating volume and there are no obvious changes apart from the patient perhaps feeling uncomfortable and restless.

- Class 2 (15–30% loss) is associated with a rise in pulse rate to >100, reduced urine output to 20–30 mL per hour, raised respiratory rate of 20–30 breaths per minute. Blood pressure is normal but pulse pressure is reduced.

- Class 3 (30–40% loss) is associated with a tachycardia of >120 bpm, reduction in both pulse pressure an blood pressure and reduction in urine output to 10–20 mL per minute.

With class 4 (>40% blood loss) the patient becomes anxious and may be confused. There is a tachycardia of >130 bpm, blood pressure and pulse pressure are low and the patient is anuric. Respiratory rate is >40 breaths per minute.

14 C

Different sutures have particular properties, which make them useful for different purposes. They can be classified into absorbable vs non-absorbable; monofilament vs multifilament and synthetic vs natural. Absorbable sutures are used for the closure of tissues that heal quickly, whereas non-absorbable ones are used for those that take longer. Monofilament sutures glide through tissues more smoothly than multifilament and are therefore useful in vascular surgery, whereas braided sutures give knots more 'hold'.

15   A

Different local anaesthetics have different maximal recommended doses. Exceeding these may result in toxicity, which presents as perioral tingling, paraesthesia, anxiety and drowsiness, and may progress to coma and CVS collapse. Use of adrenaline together with a local anaesthetic slows the systemic absorption and therefore prolongs duration of action and increases the maximum recommended dose. Lignocaine is commonly used for minor operations; bupivicaine has a longer duration of action and is used in epidural and spinal anaesthesia. Prilocaine is used in regional nerve blocks. Maximum recommended doses are: lignocaine 3 mg/kg, bupivicaine 2 mg/kg and prilocaine 6 mg/kg. The corresponding doses for preparations containing adrenaline are 5, 3 and 6 mg, respectively.

16   B

During inspiration the thorax expands causing the pleural pressure to drop resulting in air entry. The upper ribs (2–7) move with a 'pump handle' action therefore increasing the AP diameter of the thorax. The lower ribs (8–12) move with a 'bucket handle' type action which increases the lateral diameter. Movement of the ribs is brought about by contraction of the internal and external intercostal muscles. Expiration is a passive process owing to elastic recoil of the lungs. The first rib is immobile. Contraction of the diaphragm causes it to flatten and therefore increases the vertical diameter of the thorax during inspiration.

17   C

The heart is formed from a primitive heart tube, which develops five swellings: truncus arteriosus (forms aorta and pulmonary trunk and infundibulum of ventricles); bulbus cordis; ventricle; atrium; and sinus venosus (forms the smooth walled part of the atrial walls). Inside the right atrium this smooth part and a rough area (true atrium) are separated by a ridge called the crista terminalis. The sino-atrial node is situated at the top of this. Anterior cardiac veins drain directly into the right atrium. The fossa ovalis is the obliterated foramen ovale, which allows the passage of blood from the right to the left atrium in the fetus therefore bypassing the lungs. It remains patent in 10% of the population.

18   B

The subclavian vein and internal jugular veins join on each side forming the brachiocephalic veins, which then drain into the SCV. However, although there is a right brachiocephalic artery (which arises from the arch of the aorta and gives rises to the right subclavian artery and right common carotid artery), there is no corresponding left brachiocephalic artery, and the left subclavian artery and common carotid artery arise directly from the arch of the aorta. The SCV and IVC drain separately into the right atrium.

19   B

The abdominal aorta passes through the crura of the diaphragm at the level of T12 and descends to L4 where it divides into left and right common iliacs and a median sacral artery. It gives off three unpaired visceral branches (coeliac trunk at T12, superior mesenteric artery at L1 and inferior mesenteric artery at L3). There are three paired visceral branches (suprarenal vessels, renal arteries and gonadal arteries) and five paired parietal branches (to the diaphragm) and four paired lumbar arteries (to the posterior abdominal wall).

20   D

The adrenals lie within the renal fascia and receive their blood supply from the suprarenal arteries, branches of the renal arteries and branches of the inferior phrenic arteries. The kidneys are retroperitoneal organs and lie at the L2 level. The duodenum lies over the hilum of the right kidney and the small intestine lies over the inferior pole of both kidneys. Renal arteries divide into five segmental arteries with four passing anterior to the renal pelvis and one passing posteriorly.

21   C

The axilla is a space shaped like a pyramid which has anterior posterior and medial walls. The anterior wall is formed by pectoralis major and minor; the posterior wall is formed by subscapularis, latissimus dorsi and teres major and the medial wall is formed by serratus anterior and the ribs. The floor is formed by axillary fascia. The apex is formed by the first rib, clavicle and scapula.

22   A

The lower leg is divided into three compartments: anterior, posterior and lateral. The interosseous membrane running between the tibia and fibula divides the anterior and posterior compartments, while the anterior and posterior fascial septums, which both attach to the fibular, enclose the lateral compartment. The posterior compartment is further divided into deep and superficial compartments by the transverse fascia. The deep compartment contains tibialis posterior, flexor digitorum longus, flexor hallucis longus and popliteus, and the superficial compartment contains gastrocnemius, soleus and plantaris. It also contains the tibial nerve. The anterior compartment contains tibialis anterior, extensor digitorum longus, extensor hallucis longus and the deep peroneal nerve. The lateral compartment contains peroneus longus and brevis and the superficial peroneal nerve.

23   C

The femoral nerve is formed from nerve roots L2–L4 and is the nerve of the anterior thigh, it supplies psoas, iliacus, tensor fascia lata, sartorius and quadriceps femoris. It also supplies sensation to a strip of skin on the medial side of the lower leg as far as the big toe. Damage to this nerve therefore results in sensory loss in this area of skin and also loss of knee extension.

24   D

The radial nerve arises from the posterior cord of the brachial plexus and passes along the posterior aspect of the humerus in the spiral groove where it is vulnerable to damage from a fractured humerus. It then pierces the lateral intermuscular septum and divides into the posterior interosseous nerve and the superficial radial nerve at the level of the lateral epicondyle. Damage to the nerve in the spiral groove causes wrist drop but not loss of elbow extension because the nerves supplying the triceps muscle are given off more proximal to this. To also cause loss of elbow extension, damage would have to be at the level of the axilla.

25   B

The femoral canal is a space, approximately 0.5 cm in diameter, which lies between the medial aspect of the femoral sheath and the wall of the femoral vein. It allows the passage of lower limb lymphatics and allows for expansion of the femoral vessels. It also contains fat and Cloquet's node.

26   C

The parotid gland lies between the mastoid process and the sternocleidomastoid muscle posteriorly and the ramus of the mandible anteriorly. The upper pole lies between the cartilaginous part of the auditory tube and the capsule of the temporomandibular joint. The lower pole lies below and behind the angle of the mandible. The parotid duct emerges from the anterior border of the gland and pierces buccinator at the level of the 2nd upper molar tooth to enter the mouth. Structures that pass through the parotid gland are the external carotid artery (which divides within the gland into its terminal branches), retromandibular vein and facial nerve. Tumours can therefore cause a facial palsy due to nerve infiltration.

27   B

The larynx is made up of cartilages and associated ligaments, which move from the action of the laryngeal muscles. The four main cartilages are the thyroid cartilage (found at the level of C4 and a IVth arch derivative), arytenoid cartilage, cricoid cartilage (found at the level of C6 and a VIth arch derivative) and the epiglottis. All of the intrinsic muscles of the larynx except cricothyroid are supplied by the recurrent laryngeal nerve. Cricothyroid is supplied by the superior laryngeal nerve. The actions of the intrinsic muscles open the cords (posterior cricoarytenoids), close the larynx during swallowing (lateral cricoarytenoids) and alter the tension of the cords to change pitch during speech (thyroarytenoids and cricothyroids).

28   E

Important surface landmarks in the abdomen include: liver, from the nipple line to the 10th rib; gallbladder, at 9th costal cartilage midclavicular line; kidney, superior pole at the level of the 12th rib posteriorly; pancreas, at L1; spleen, overlying the 9th, 10th and 11th ribs posteriorly. The transpyloric plane of Addison lies midway between the suprasternal notch and the pubis at the level of L1.

29   C

The diaphragm arises from the six lower costal cartilages laterally, xiphoid anteriorly, arcuate ligaments and crura posteriorly. The left crus arises from the lumbar vertebrae L1–2 and the right one arises from L1–3. The following structures pierce the diaphragm: at T8 – left phrenic nerve and IVC; at T10 – oesophagus and vagi; at T12 aorta and thoracic duct. It is also pierced by the splanchnic nerves and sympathetic chain.

30   A

The bladder is covered only on its upper aspect by peritoneum. Its muscular wall is formed by the detrusor muscle and it is lined by transitional epithelium. The triangular shaped area at the bladder base, which lies between the two ureteric orifices, is the trigone. The detrusor muscle is supplied by parasympathetic fibres, which cause contraction, and sympathetic fibres, which cause relaxation. It has an internal sphincter formed by smooth muscle and an external sphincter, which lies below the prostate in the male. The blood supply comes from the superior and inferior vesical arteries, which are branches of the internal iliac artery.

31   B

Full thickness burns are typically black/white in colour and insensate. They exhibit minimal healing and usually require skin grafting. They do not blanch when touched. In contrast superficial burns are pink and painful and often associated with blistering. 100% repair after 2 weeks but healing may be associated with pigment changes.

32   D

Wallace's Rule of Nines is used to calculate the percentage body area involved. It works by attributing a percentage to a body part: Head = 9%; arm (each) = 9%; legs (each) 18% (9% each surface); trunk 36%; perineum 1%; palm 1.25%. Calculating the percentage burn helps to guide fluid resuscitation – intravenous fluids are essential when this exceeds 15%.

33   D

The obturator nerve supplies the muscles in the medial compartment of the thigh and arises from the lumbar plexus (L1–4 ventral rami). It also supplies sensation to a patch of skin on the medial aspect of the thigh. Irritation of this nerve by pelvic pathology may result in pain in this distribution because the lateral pelvic peritoneum is supplied by the obturator nerve as it passes through the pelvis.

34   C

Mechanical ventilation is used for unconscious patients and also to provide oxygen therapy where other methods have failed. It is unfortunately associated with several complications. As a result of the positive pressure required there is a risk of barotrauma (pneumothorax, pneumomediastinum, pneumoperitoneum and surgical emphysema) and venous return is reduced, which decreases cardiac filling. Ventilation can also cause gastric dilatation and ileus, and long-term use can lead to atrophy of the respiratory muscles. Infection and airway damage are other risks.

35　D

ARDS is a specific disease of the lungs characterised by hypoxaemia, alveolar inflammation and oedema and pulmonary fibrosis. Clinically the patient has a raised respiratory rate; cyanosis and arterial blood gases show hypercapnia. Lung compliance is greatly reduced, therefore increasing the work required. There are certain criteria that need to be met in order to make a diagnosis of ARDS. These are: severe hypoxaemia (PaO$_2$/FiO$_2$ of <27), pulmonary infiltrates on chest X-ray, pulmonary artery wedge pressure of <18mmHg (therefore non-cardiogenic pulmonary oedema) and a recognised cause. There are a variety of causes including pancreatitis, sepsis, DIC, burns and aspiration.

36　C

The cause of oliguria can be determined by looking at urine and serum samples. This helps to differentiate between renal and pre-renal causes. Pre-renal renal failure will have low urinary sodium (<20 mmol/L) and a serum osmolarity ratio of >1.2, serum creatinine ratio of >40 and a high urine osmolarity of >500. Conversely, renal causes have high urinary sodium of >40 mmol/L, serum osmolarity ratio of <1.2, serum creatinine ratio <20 and an osmolarity of <350.

37　E

Brainstem death is defined as irreversible cessation of brainstem function and is diagnosed by carrying out specific tests. These tests cannot be carried out if the patient is hypothermic (<35°C) has had depressant drugs or has metabolic derangements. The patient must be in an apnoeic coma requiring ventilation and have a known cause of brain damage. The tests are designed to test the cranial nerves and are: papillary response, corneal reflex, pain reflex (facial nerve distribution), caloric test (instillation of ice cold water into ear and looking for nystagmus towards that side), gag reflex and apnoea test.

38   D

SIRS involves the systemic activation of the acute phase response following an insult. It is defined by the presence of two or more of the following: tachycardia of >90 bpm, respiratory rate of >20 breaths per minute or $PaCO_2$ of <4.3 kPa, temperature of >38°C or <36°C and white blood count of >12 or <4 × 10^9/L.

39   B

Tumour markers are substances found in the blood associated with certain cancers. They are used in diagnosis, surveillance and staging. Non-seminomatous germ cell tumours of the testis are associated with a raised alpha fetoprotein and raised beta human chorionic gonadotrophin (HCG). PSA is a tumour marker for prostate cancer but is also elevated in BPH and prostatitis. Ca125 is mainly elevated in mucinous ovarian carcinoma but is also seen in breast and pancreatic cancer. CEA is a marker for colorectal cancer as well as ovarian and breast cancer. Ca19–9 is sometimes elevated in pancreatic cancer and advanced colorectal cancer.

40   C

MEN is a familial autosomal dominant disorder. There are two types: MEN 1 (pituitary adenomas, pancreatic islet tumours, hyperplasia of the parathyroids and tumours of the adrenal cortex) and MEN 2, which is further subdivided into MEN 2a (medullary thyroid carcinoma, phaeochromocytoma, parathyroid adenoma/hyperplasia) and MEN 2b (parathyroid tumours, medullary thyroid carcinoma, phaeochromocytoma, multiple mucosal neuromas and Marfanoid habitus). MEN syndromes can be picked up by genetic screening techniques.

41   A

Squamous cell carcinoma is a malignant tumour of epidermal keratinocytes and is most commonly found on areas of the body that have been exposed to the sun. Surgery should achieve a 1–2 cm clearance margin. This is in contrast to the management of basal cell carcinoma (0.5 cm clearance margin) and malignant melanoma, which is based on clinical appearance (impalpable – 1 cm; palpable – 2 cm; nodular – 3 cm).

42   C

Duct ectasia is dilatation and inflammation of the mammary ducts and commonly affects middle-aged women. It usually presents with tenderness, erythema and a green/brown nipple discharge. Discharge can be physiological in lactation, pregnancy, and following mechanical stimulation. Blood-stained discharge is a worrying sign and may indicate carcinoma of duct papilloma. Breast abscess do not tend to present with nipple discharge. They usually present with pain, fever, swelling and erythema.

43   C

Genetic factors are an important consideration in breast cancer as the BRCA 1 and 2 genes are implicated in 2% of cases. It may also be associated with genetic syndromes such as Li–Fraumeni syndrome. Other risk factors include advanced age (risk rises linearly with age), hyperplasia with atypia of breast tissue, nulliparity, early menarche/late menopause and obesity.

44   A

Cytology reports grade samples according to the cellular appearances by a 5-point system. C1 = inadequate sample, C2 = benign, C3 = equivocal, C4 = suspicious for malignancy and C5 = malignant. Fine needle aspiration cytology (FNAC) forms part of the triple assessment for suspected breast cancer along with clinical examination and imaging (mammogram or ultrasound).

45   D

Blood flows in an 'outward to inward' direction towards the myocardium. During systole, contraction of the ventricles causes compression of the coronary vessels, reducing or even reversing blood flow. This means that it is in diastole when the most blood reaches the myocardium of the left ventricle. Changes in myocardial activity and demand result in release of mediators, which autoregulate the coronary flow according to need. The right coronary artery, which arises from the right aortic sinus, mainly supplies the right ventricle. The left coronary artery, which arises from the left aortic sinus, supplies the left ventricle. Blood supply to the atria is variable. The interventricular septum is supplied by both arteries.

46   D

Prostate cancer is staged using the TMN system. Staging often determines the management plan. T1 disease is present when the tumour is not palpable or visible and is picked up on examination of the chips obtained at TURP. T2 disease is when the tumour is confined to the prostate and can be further subdivided into 2a (one lobe) and 2b (two lobes). T3 disease is when there is extension through the capsule, with T3a being extracapsular disease and T3b being invasion into the seminal vesicles. T4 is when the tumour is fixed or is invading into adjacent structures. In this example, the patient has T3b disease, which would be treated with hormone therapy and radiotherapy.

47   B

Mitomycin C is an agent instilled intravesically for the treatment of superficial transitional cell carcinoma of the bladder, to prevent a recurrence. Finasteride is a 5-α reductase inhibitor. By blocking the action of 5-α reductase, it reduces the formation of dihydrotestosterone, therefore reducing the stimulatory effect this has on prostate gland growth. Oxybutynin is an anticholinergic agent used in the management of detrusor instability. Tamsulosin is an alpha adrenergic blocker used in the management of BPH. It causes smooth muscle relaxation of prostate and bladder neck, therefore improving urine flow rates. Flutamine is used in the management of prostate cancer. It is an antiandrogen and works by preventing testosterone from causing growth of the tumour.

48   C

A hydrocele is an abnormal collection of fluid in the tunica vaginalis surrounding the testis or spermatic cord. They occur in males of any age but are most common at extreme ends of the age spectrum. They can present from birth owing to the fact, that during descent of the testis from the abdomen to the scrotum, a sac of peritoneum is pulled along, which envelops the testis and epididymis creating a tubular communication between the abdomen and the tunica vaginalis of the scrotum. Usually the part surrounding the spermatic cord obliterates, therefore closing off this communication. If it does not, a congenital hydrocele is formed where fluid accumulates within the patent processus vaginalis and around the testis. If the processus vaginalis obliterates at the level of the deep inguinal ring, the resulting hydrocele is an infantile hydrocele. If fluid is present in the tunica vaginalis surrounding the testis but not the spermatic cord, this is a vaginal hydrocele. A hydrocele of the cord is formed when the distal portion of the processus vaginalis closes, the midportion remains patent and fluid filled and the proximal portion may be open or closed. In older men, an increase in the production of serous fluid by the tunica vaginalis (eg owing to infection, trauma or tumour) can result in a hydrocele. In 10% of cases a testicular tumour is associated with a hydrocele.

49   E

These symptoms are most likely due to a testicular torsion. This has to be considered a surgical emergency as the longer this is left, the higher the chance of testicular infarction. The purpose of surgery is to correct the torsion in the affected testis and to anchor the other testis to prevent future torsion. This can be achieved via a transverse incision over the testis or via a small midline incision in the scrotal raphe. If the testis is found to be clearly necrotic, it should be removed.

50   C

TURP is performed by passing a resectoscope through the urethra into the bladder and using a wire loop to pass electrical current to resect the prostate gland. It is a relatively safe procedure (mortality <0.25%) but is associated with certain complications. These include urinary incontinence (2–4%), erectile dysfunction (5%), urethral stricture (5%), retrograde ejaculation (65%) and increase risk of MI. In addition there is the risk of developing TUR syndrome, which is due to the absorption of irrigation fluid into the body. This presents with hypotension, bradycardia, nausea and vomiting and collapse. Blood tests show hyponatraemia.

51   E

The rotator cuff is a ring of muscles that surrounds and strengthens the shoulder joint, but is deficient inferiorly. They attach at the level of the anatomical neck of the humerus. Specifically the attachments are: subscapularis to the lesser tuberosity; supraspinatus, teres minor and infraspinatus to the greater tuberosity (in that order from above down). As well as moving the shoulder joint they also act as a muscular support. Supraspinatus runs thorough a tunnel formed by the acromion and the coraco-acromial ligament and its tendon is fused to the capsule of the shoulder joint.

52   C

Paraumbilical hernias occur just above and just below the umbilicus and are more commonly seen in women. They are acquired, and predisposing factors are obesity and multiple pregnancies. They are at high risk of strangulation as the neck is usually narrow. A hernia that contains a strangulated Meckel's diverticulum is known as a Littre's hernia and can progress to gangrene, suppuration and formation of a local fistula. Hernias that present below and lateral to the pubic tubercle are femoral hernias as opposed to inguinal hernias, which present above and medial to the pubic tubercle. Hernias that appear spontaneously just superior to the iliac crest are most likely to be lumbar hernias. They occur through the lumbar triangle of Petit formed by the iliac crest, posterior external oblique and anterior latissimus dorsi. Spigelian hernias present through the linea semilunaris at the lateral border of the rectus sheath. They occur at the point where the posterior rectus sheath becomes deficient posteriorly.

53   C

Radiotherapy uses ionising radiation to kill cells. Doses are given at intervals allowing the normal tissues to recover, but preventing the malignant cells, which take longer to regenerate from growing. It works by damaging DNA through release of kinetic energy and can be administered through a variety of methods including electrons, protons, neutrons, X-rays and gamma rays. The success of radiotherapy treatment is dependent on the radiosensitivity of the tumour (for example seminoma is very radiosensitive) and the tolerance of the surrounding tissue, as this can limit the amount of radiotherapy administered. It can be given as a primary treatment, adjuvant and neo-adjuvant therapy and palliative treatment. Palliation of bone pain can be a single treatment. Complications include ulceration, bleeding, delayed wound healing and lymphoedema.

54   D

Lung function tests are useful pre-operatively as they provide the anaesthetist with information about lung function and capacity. Lung volumes vary with sex/height but not weight. The tidal volume is the amount of air moved into/out of the lung during quiet respiration. The amount of air that can be inspired on top of this is the inspiratory reserve volume, and the amount of air that can be forcibly expired on top of the tidal volume is the expiratory reserve volume. Air left in the lung at the end of a maximal expiration is the residual volume. The residual volume together with the expiratory reserve volume is the functional residual capacity. This is important as it is the volume in which gas exchange takes place. Total lung capacity is the sum of the residual volume and the vital capacity, which is the volume expired after a maximum inspiration.

55   C

Arterial ulcers are typically found at the 'pressure points' of the foot, ie tips of the toes, heel and over the malleoli. They are painful and have a 'punched out' appearance. Poor blood flow to the feet is associated with venous guttering and this can be seen in association with arterial ulcers. Conversely, venous ulcers are usually found around the gaiter area, have sloping edges and are associated with skin changes such as haemosiderin deposition and lipodermatosclerosis (skin induration due to fibrosis of subcutaneous fat).

56   D

Carotid endarterectomy is a procedure carried out to remove an atherosclerotic plaque from the carotid artery in patients who have suffered TIAs or CVAs. The procedure is usually restricted to those who have 70% stenosis of the artery or above because it is at this point that the benefits outweigh the risks of the operation. It involves making an incision in the neck and locating the carotid artery, clamping it above and below the stenosis, creating a bypass for the blood to flow to the head during the operation and incising the artery to remove the plaque. The major risks involved include CVA (1–3%), MI (the most major cause of mortality), glossopharyngeal nerve injury and re-accumulation of the atheroma.

57   C

Arterial stenoses that are short and localised in nature are amenable to treatment with percutaneous balloon angioplasty. Much better long-term results are achieved if the lesion is present in a proximal vessel such as the SFA. The procedure is carried out by the Seldinger technique, where a flexible guide-wire is passed across the stenosis and then a catheter with a plastic inflatable balloon is passed across it. The balloon is dilated when it reaches the stenosis, widening the vessel.

58   B

Intermittent claudication is a pain in muscle owing to ischaemia brought on by exercise and relieved by rest. The site of the pain often indicates the area of stenosis: for example calf pain suggests superficial femoral artery, thigh suggests external iliac artery and buttock pain suggests common iliac artery. Occlusion of the aorto-iliac region associated with buttock claudication and impotence is known as Leriche's syndrome.

C   59

Elective surgery is normally carried out for AAA only if the patient is relatively fit and has an aneurysm >5.5 cm in diameter, as the mortality for the operation is 5%. Endoluminal stenting is a relatively new alternative that can be used to treat infrarenal aneurysms. Overall mortality in ruptured aneurysms is 75% and unstable patients should proceed to urgent surgery. Ultrasound scan or CT scan can aid diagnosis, and regular ultrasound scans are a means of carrying out regular surveillance of aneurysms not large enough to require surgery. Thrombus formation within aneurysms may lead to distal emboli. AAAs are much more common in men.

60   D

Lymphoedema is an abnormal collection of tissue fluid from defective lymphatics, and may be either primary or secondary in nature. Secondary causes include infection, malignancy and radiotherapy. Surgery is rarely used to treat it and management is usually conservative with compression stockings, intermittent mechanical compression and treatment of cellulitis when it occurs. Ulceration is not commonly seen with primary lymphoedema.

61   C

Bone cysts are common benign fluid-containing lesions that usually occur in the metaphysic of long bones. Half of all bone cysts present as pathological fractures and most occur in children aged 4–10. Bone metastases usually present with pain, although occurrence of a pathological fracture may be the first presentation. Osteosarcoma has a bimodal distribution with 75% of those affected being aged between 10 and 25 years. The remainder are elderly with a history of Paget's disease. It typically presents with a painful mass, most commonly affecting the lower femur and arising from the medullary cavity. Chondrosarcomas can present de novo or from malignant transformation of a benign cartilage tumour such an osteochondroma. They usually affect middle-aged or elderly people. Ewing's sarcoma usually affects young people aged between 5 and 15 years. It presents as a lytic lesion, which causes a periosteal reaction giving it a characteristic 'onion skin' appearance.

62   E

Osteomyelitis is characterised by pain and swelling over the affected part and a fever. Bacteria may enter the bone via direct inoculation or haematogenous spread. People most susceptible are those with diabetes and immunosuppression. Radiological changes do not usually appear until 10 days after onset and consist of soft tissue swelling and sclerotic bone changes with periosteal elevation. The most likely causative organism in this case is *Staphylococcus aureus*. In young children, *Haemophilus influenzae* may also be a cause. *Salmonella* can cause osteomyelitis in sickle cell patients.

63   D

Carpal tunnel syndrome is due to compression of the median nerve within the carpal tunnel, which is itself made up of the carpal bones and the transverse carpal ligament. It may be idiopathic or associated with pregnancy, rheumatoid arthritis, diabetes or hypothyroidism. It typically presents with pain and paraesthesia over the thumb and lateral two fingers, which is worse at night. There may be associated wasting of the thenar muscles. Tinnel's test involves reproduction of symptoms on tapping over the carpal tunnel whereas Phalen's test involves reproduction of symptoms on flexing the wrist.

64   D

Characteristic radiological features of osteoarthritis are bone cysts, subchondral sclerosis, osteophytes, reduced joint space and joint effusion. In contrast, features of rheumatoid arthritis are periarticular soft tissue swelling, loss of joint space, bony erosions, juxta-articular osteoporosis and pseudocysts.

65   C

The popliteal fossa is a diamond-shaped area on the back of the knee. It is bounded superiorly by biceps femoris (laterally) and semimembranosus (medially) and the two heads of gastrocnemius (inferiorly). The roof is formed by deep fascia pierced by the short saphenous vein. It contains the branches of the sciatic nerve (tibial and common peroneal nerves), the popliteal vein and artery. The deepest structure is the artery. The common peroneal nerve lies laterally and winds around the head of the fibula, whereas the tibial nerve lies medially.

66   D

The brachial plexus is made up of five nerve roots (C5–T1), which then form trunks in the posterior triangle of the neck. C6 and C7 join to form the superior trunk, C7 continues as the middle trunk and C8 and T1 from the inferior trunk. The trunks divide into anterior and posterior divisions and then combine to form lateral posterior and medial cords. The cords divide to form the main nerves: musculocutaneous nerve (lateral cord), median nerve (lateral and medial cords), axillary nerve (posterior cord), radial nerve (posterior cord) and ulnar nerve (medial cord). There are several branches arising from the roots, trunks and cords. For example: the long thoracic nerve, which supplies serratus anterior, arises from nerve roots C5–C7; the thoracodorsal nerve, which supplies latissimus dorsi, arises from the posterior cord, whereas the nerve to subscapularis arises from the posterior cord.

67   B

A posterior dislocation of the hip causes the leg to appear shortened and internally rotated. In 20% of fracture dislocations of the hip, the sciatic nerve is damaged. This results in paralysis of the hamstrings and all the flexors and extensors below the knee. Also, all of the skin below the knee loses its sensation apart from the areas supplied by the saphenous and posterior cutaneous nerve of the thigh (medial and upper posterior calf respectively).

68   D

Supraspinatus tendonitis is usually caused by vigorous exercise in people over 40 years. They present with a 'painful arc' of shoulder movement when the arm passes through 60–120 degrees of abduction. In contrast supraspinatus rupture makes active abduction impossible, although there is a full range of passive movement. Frozen shoulder occurs as a result of degenerative changes of the rotator cuff. Pain due to this causes the patient to hold the shoulder still and adhesions form, which limit movement even more until only scapular movement remains. Rupture of the long head of biceps usually occurs in a previously diseased tendon and causes pain, tenderness and bunching up of the muscle in the lower arm.

69   E

Fractured neck of the femur is unfortunately a common injury in the elderly and mortality is in the region of 30% at 6 months. Patients usually present with a history of a fall and then inability to weight bear on the affected side. On inspection the affected leg is shortened and externally rotated. The way in which fractured neck of femur is managed is dictated by the blood supply to the femoral head. A significant amount of the blood supply comes from the retinacular vessels, which pass proximally within the joint capsule. These vessels are therefore disrupted in intracapsular (subcapital) fractures. Undisplaced subcapital fractures have a good chance of maintaining the blood supply as there is minimal disruption of the capsule. They can generally be treated with insertion of cannulated screws. If they are displaced (ie Garden III and IV), there is a high risk of developing avascular necrosis of the femoral head and so hemiarthroplasty is the preferred management.

70   C

The safest operation to carry out in these circumstances, where a patient is unstable and the operating field is highly contaminated, is a Hartman's operation, where the affected segment of colon is excised and the proximal end is brought out as an end colostomy. The rectal stump is closed and left inside or alternatively may be brought out as a mucous fistula. It is possible then to rejoin the two ends of bowel once the patient is in a more stable state and infection has settled to allow optimum conditions for forming an anastomosis.

71   C

Gastrectomy is an effective treatment for gastric carcinoma but is associated with possible long-term complications. Dumping syndrome is due to the fact that food and liquid passes too quickly into the small intestine causing abdominal cramps, diarrhoea, dizziness, sweating, nausea and vomiting. It is thought to be due to accelerated gastric emptying of hyperosmolar contents into the small bowel. This leads to fluid shifts from the intravascular compartment into the bowel lumen. It is often relieved by dietary changes. Another possible problem is vitamin B_{12} deficiency: the stomach is where intrinsic factor is secreted by the parietal cells and also stomach acid helps to release vitamin B_{12} from ingested food. Bolus obstruction can occur from the relative reduction in volume of the small intestine compared with the stomach. Hypocalcaemia can also occur postgastrectomy and is due to increased transit time and therefore reduced time over which absorption can occur. Because of this malabsorption, weight loss is commonly seen postgastrectomy.

72   B

The jejunum forms the upper 2/5ths of the small bowel whereas the ileum forms the lower 3/5ths. There are certain anatomical differences between the two. Compared with the ileum, the jejunum has a thicker wall, more valvulae conniventes, a greater number of villi and a wider lumen. There is also a difference in the arrangement of the blood vessels in the small bowel mesentery. The ileal vessels form complex branching arcades before reaching the bowel, whereas the jejunal vessels have a much simpler arrangement.

73   B

Ulcerative colitis is a disease of the mucosa lining the rectum that spreads proximally in a continuous manner to involve a variable proportion of the colon. In a few cases the terminal ileum is involved and this is termed backwash ileitis. Even less commonly, the perianal region may be involved, although this is much more common in Crohn's disease. Unlike Crohn's disease, which is transmural, the inflammation in UC is restricted to the mucosa causing oedema, ulceration and pseudopolyps. Granulomas are a typical feature of Crohn's disease but not of UC.

74   B

Diverticular disease can cause bowel obstruction, either as a result of repeated episodes of inflammation, which causes fibrosis and strictures, or due to a diverticular mass, which obstructs the lumen. Similarly an adenocarcinoma of the bowel, particularly if it is annular in nature, can also cause obstruction. Crohn's disease causes transmural inflammation and this also results in stricturing. Gallstones may erode into the duodenum causing a gallstone ileus. Angioplasia is a vascular malformation that can result in PR bleeding, most commonly in the elderly. It does not cause obstruction.

75   C

Constipation can occur for many different reasons. Volvulus is a twisting of a loop of bowel around its mesenteric axis resulting in partial or complete obstruction and therefore constipation. It also causes abdominal pain and nausea and vomiting. Painful anal conditions, such as anal fissure, can also result in constipation as the patient is reluctant to pass stool. CVA together with Parkinson's disease and Hirschsprung's disease causes adynamic bowel and therefore constipation. Drugs such as opiate analgesics, aspirin and anticonvulsants are also known causes. Digoxin is known to cause diarrhoea.

76   E

Inflammatory bowel disease is associated with several extraintestinal manifestations. These include erythema nodosum, pyoderma gangrenosum, uveitis, iritis, episcleritis, seronegative arthritis, sclerosing cholangitis and cirrhosis. Rarely systemic amyloidosis may occur, but sarcoidosis is not a known association.

77   D

The Glasgow scale is one of the scoring systems used to determine the severity of an attack of pancreatitis. The criteria used are: age >55, WBC >15 × 10^9, blood glucose >10 mmol/L, serum urea >16 mmol/L, PaO$_2$ <60 mmHg, serum calcium <2.0 mmol/L, albumin <32 g/L, LDH >600 units/L, AST/ALT >600 U/L. The other scoring system in use is Ranson's criteria.

78   D

Early splenomegaly is usually asymptomatic but, as the spleen increases in size, it may cause abdominal discomfort and early satiety from gastric compression. It may be the result of several different aetiologies. These include infection (eg CMV, malaria/TB/syphilis), autoimmune disease (eg rheumatoid arthritis and SLE), haematological disorders (eg leukaemia, lymphoma, polycythaemia and haemolytic anaemia) and other causes such as amyloidosis.

79   C

Carotid body tumours present as masses adjacent to the hyoid bone and anterior to the sternocleidomastoid. They are typically pulsatile, compressible and smooth with mobility in the horizontal but not vertical plane. Approximately 5% are malignant. Cystic hygromas are congenital lymphatic malformations situated at the root of the neck and are present at birth in 50% of neonates. Sternocleidomastoid tumours are usually found in the neonatal period and are located at the junction between the upper and middle thirds of the muscle. They tend to disappear with age. Laryngoceles are saccules that become expanded with air, often after straining. Dermoid cysts may be congenital or acquired. Congenital cysts are commonly located on the head or neck and acquired cysts are most commonly caused when a piece of skin is implanted into the dermis secondary to trauma.

80   B

Thyroid surgery is associated with several complications. Hypothyroidism is an expected result and requires replacement with oral thyroxine. Haematoma formation can occur and, if it becomes enlarged, can compress the trachea requiring urgent evacuation. Laryngeal oedema can be caused by trauma sustained during surgery and may make airway management difficult. There is a risk to the recurrent laryngeal and superior laryngeal nerves during thyroid surgery. Damage to the superior laryngeal nerve results in a monotonous voice because of paralysis of the cricothyroid muscle. Hypocalcaemia can result from inadvertent damage to the parathyroid glands and requires oral replacement.

81   B

Pruritus ani is a common condition, which may be due to a variety of causes. Men are more commonly affected and symptoms worsen during hot weather and at night. Causes include skin diseases (eg eczema and psoriasis), general medical diseases (eg diabetes, myeloproliferative disorders, lymphoma and obstructive jaundice), perianal disease (eg anal fissure and Crohn's disease) and local irritants such as mucus and sweat. Often an 'itch/scratch' cycle is set up and so symptoms can persist even when the cause has been eradicated.

82   C

The parotid gland is known as the 80% gland because: 80% of salivary tumours are found in the parotid. Of these, 80% are benign in nature and 80% of these are pleomorphic adenomas. Another benign tumour of the parotid is an adenolymphoma. Adenocarcinoma of the parotid makes up 3% of all parotid tumours. It may infiltrate the facial nerve, which runs through the parotid, causing a facial palsy. Management is by parotidectomy, with the aim of preserving the facial nerve if it is not involved. Damage to the innervation of the parotid gland during surgery can result in Frey's syndrome. This is due to inappropriate regeneration of parasympathetic nerve fibres, which stimulate the sweat glands of overlying skin resulting in gustatory sweating. 15% of salivary gland neoplasms are located in the submandibular gland.

83   C

Anaplastic thyroid tumours are most commonly found in elderly females and present as a rapidly expanding neck mass. 50% present with distant metastases and prognosis is poor. Radiotherapy can be used for palliation of local disease whereas chemotherapy has a role in treating distant metastases. In early anaplastic cancer, the outlook is better and may be treated by surgery followed by radiotherapy.

84   C

Cushing's syndrome is a disease caused by an excess of cortisol production or by excessive use of cortisol or other similar steroid (glucocorticoid) hormones. It can be diagnosed either by measuring 24-hour urinary free cortisol or by an overnight dexamethasone suppression test, which fails to suppress morning cortisol levels in affected patients. Cushing's disease is the name given to a type of Cushing's syndrome caused by too much ACTH production in the pituitary. Phaeochromocytomas are tumours of the adrenal medulla arising from chromaffin cells and secreting excess catecholamines. Vanillylmandelic acid (VMA) is a breakdown product of catecholamines and therefore urinary levels become elevated and are used as a diagnostic test. Conn's syndrome is caused by an aldosterone-secreting adrenocortical adenoma and causes raised plasma aldosterone. Addison's disease is often associated with other autoimmune disorders and is characterised by low serum cortisol. It can be investigated for by using the short synacthen test, which doesn't cause a rise in plasma cortisol in affected patients whereas it does in unaffected people. Congenital adrenal hyperplasia occurs as a result of 2,1-hydroxylase deficiency.

85   C

First-line treatment for thyrotoxicosis disease is carbimazole. In certain individuals it has the unfortunate side effect of agranulocytosis and so propythiouracil is used instead. This is also the drug of choice in pregnancy as it is protein bound and therefore less likely to cross the placenta. Radio-iodide ablation is safe for patients in whom medical management has failed and who are not planning on becoming pregnant during treatment. Surgery for thyroid disorders is carried out for cosmesis, compression symptoms, retrostenal extension and carcinoma.

86   C

The muscles involved in movement of the eye are lateral rectus, medial rectus, superior rectus, inferior rectus, superior oblique and inferior oblique. All, apart from inferior oblique, arise from a fibrous ring. Lateral rectus is supplied by cranial nerve VI, superior oblique by cranial nerve IV and all the others by cranial nerve II. The orbit is made up of several bones with both wings of the sphenoid forming the posterior wall. The frontal bone forms the superior part, the lacrimal and ethmoid bones the medial part, the maxilla the inferior part and the zygoma the lateral part.

87   B

The majority of laryngeal cancers are squamous cell carcinomas. Staging and management is dependant on the location and extent of the tumour. In this case the tumour is limited to the vocal cord and there is no evidence of spread, making it a T1 tumour. This can be treated by either radiotherapy or endoscopic resection. In the case of this woman who is a singer, radiotherapy is the preferred option as there is less risk of vocal cord damage.

88   B

The thyroid is made up of two lobes connected by an isthmus that overlies the 2nd and 3rd tracheal rings. Occasionally there may be a pyramidal lobe. It obtains its blood supply from the superior thyroid artery (branch of the external carotid), which supplies the upper pole and the inferior thyroid artery (branch of the thyrocervical trunk of the subclavian artery), which supplies the lower pole and posterior part. In approximately 10% of the population there is an additional artery, the thyroid ima artery (arising from the arch of the aorta or bracheocephalic artery), which supplies the isthmus. It is drained by three veins: superior thyroid draining the upper pole, middle thyroid vein draining the lateral aspects, and inferior thyroid vein draining the lower pole. Whereas the superior and middle veins drain into the internal jugular vein, the inferior thyroid veins drain into the brachiocephalic veins.

89   C

The spleen has a significant immune function and so this is therefore impaired following splenectomy. Specifically there is a lack of splenic macrophages to clear opsonised micro-organisms and this can result in severe post-splenectomy sepsis. This most commonly affects younger patients in the first few months following splenectomy, although can occur several years later. The organisms that cause most concern are the encapsulated organisms such as *Streptococcus pneumoniae*, *Neisseria meningitidis* and *Haemophilus influenzae* B. People undergoing elective splenectomy should be immunised with the relevant vaccines preferably at least 20 weeks prior to operation. They should also be started on a prophylactic dose of penicillin V.

90   C

Extradural haematomas usually follow a blow to the head in the region of the pterion, which is where the middle meningeal artery runs in the extradural space. This results in rupture of the artery and an extradural bleed. After an initial period of concussion, there is a lucid interval while the haematoma is expanding. At the point when the haematoma can no longer be accommodated, the intracranial pressure rises and coning may occur. Management is by formation of a Burr hole to drain the haematoma.

Index